MOSBY'S

Pharmacology Memory NoteCards

Visual, Mnemonic, & Memory Aids for Nurses

JoAnn Zerwekh, MSN, EdD, RN
President/CEO
Nursing Education Consultants
Chandler, Arizona
Nursing Faculty—Online Campus
University of Phoenix
Phoenix, Arizona

CJ Miller, BSN, RN
Illustrator
Cedar Rapids, Iowa

REVIEWED BY

Pamela Harvey, MSN, BSN, ASN, RN, BLS
Instructor
Medical Assistant Program
Bradford Union Career Technical Center
Starke, Florida

Robin Ye, RPh, PharmD, BCPS, BLS
Clinical Pharmacist
NorthShore University HealthSystem
Glenbrook Hospital
Glenview, Illinois

ELSEVIER

ELSEVIER

3251 Riverport Lane
St. Louis, Missouri 63043

MOSBY'S PHARMACOLOGY MEMORY NOTECARDS: VISUAL, MNEMONIC, AND MEMORY AIDS FOR NURSES, FIFTH EDITION

ISBN: 978-0-323-54951-6

NOTICES

Knowledge and best practice in this field are constantly changing. As new research and experience broaden our understanding, changes in research methods, professional practices, or medical treatment may become necessary. Practitioners and researchers must always rely on their own experience and knowledge in evaluating and using any information, methods, compounds, or experiments described herein. In using such information or methods they should be mindful of their own safety and the safety of others, including parties for whom they have a professional responsibility.

With respect to any drug or pharmaceutical products identified, readers are advised to check the most current information provided (i) on procedures featured or (ii) by the manufacturer of each product to be administered, to verify the recommended dose or formula, the method and duration of administration, and contraindications. It is the responsibility of the practitioners, relying on their own experience and knowledge of the patient, to make diagnoses, to determine dosages and the best treatment for each individual patient, and to take all appropriate safety precautions.

To the fullest extent of the law, neither the Publisher nor the authors, contributors, or editors assume any liability for any injury and/or damage to persons or property as a matter of products' liability, negligence or otherwise, or from any use or operation of any methods, products, instructions, or ideas contained in the material herein.

International Standard Book Number: 978-0-323-54951-6

Senior Content Strategist: Jamie Blum
Content Development Manager: Lisa Newton
Content Development Specialist: Laurel Shea
Publishing Services Manager: Jeff Patterson
Senior Book Designer: Amy Buxton
Cover Art: CJ Miller

Printed in China
Last digit is the print number: 9 8 7 6 5 4 3 2 1

ADMINISTRATION

ANALGESICS AND NSAIDs

ANTIBIOTICS/ANTIVIRALS

ANTICOAGULANTS AND HEMATINICS

CARDIAC

CNS

DIURETICS

ENDOCRINE

GASTROINTESTINAL

MISCELLANEOUS

MUSCULOSKELETAL

PSYCHIATRIC

PULMONARY

REPRODUCTIVE/OB

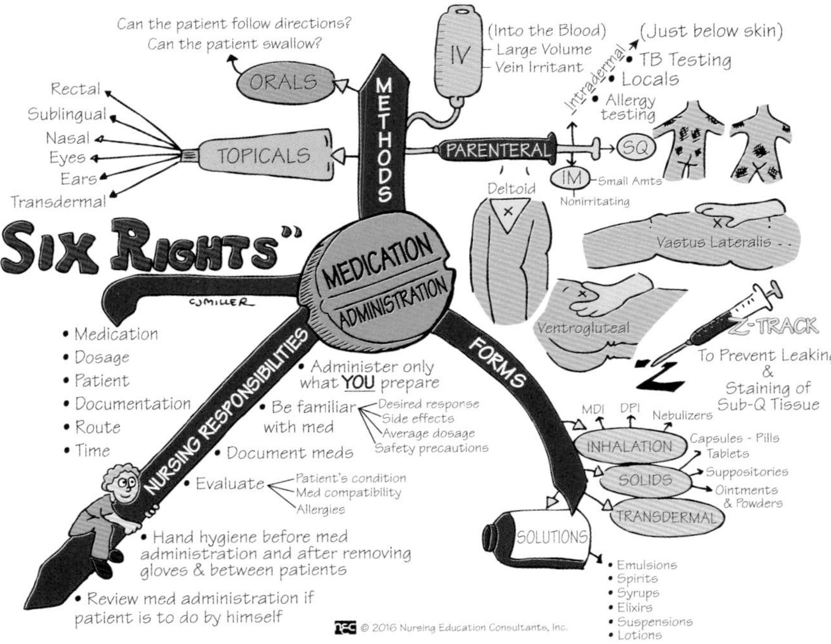
"SIX RIGHTS"
• Medication
• Dosage
• Patient
• Documentation
• Route
• Time
CJMILLER
MEDICATION
ADMINISTRATION
METHODS
ORALS
Can the patient follow directions?
Can the patient swallow?
TOPICALS
Rectal
Sublingual
Nasal
Eyes
Ears
Transdermal
PARENTERAL
IV
(Into the Blood)
Large Volume
Vein Irritant
Intradermal
(Just below skin)
• TB Testing
• Locals
• Allergy testing
SQ
Small Amts
IM
Nonirritating
Deltoid
Vastus Lateralis
Ventrogluteal
Z-TRACK
To Prevent Leaking & Staining of Sub-Q Tissue
FORMS
MDI
DPI
Nebulizers
INHALATION
Capsules - Pills
Tablets
SOLIDS
Suppositories
Ointments & Powders
TRANSDERMAL
SOLUTIONS
• Emulsions
• Spirits
• Syrups
• Elixirs
• Suspensions
• Lotions
NURSING RESPONSIBILITIES
• Administer only what YOU prepare
• Be familiar with med
Desired response
Side effects
Average dosage
Safety precautions
• Document meds
• Evaluate
Patient's condition
Med compatibility
Allergies
• Hand hygiene before med administration and after removing gloves & between patients
• Review med administration if patient is to do by himself
© 2016 Nursing Education Consultants, Inc.

What You Need to Know

Medication Administration

SIX RIGHTS OF MEDICATION ADMINISTRATION

- Medication
- Patient
- Route
- Dosage
- Time
- Documentation

ROUTES OF ADMINISTRATION

- Enteral or oral (most common)—ingested into gastrointestinal tract
- Parenteral—injected into blood or body tissues (intravenous [IV], intramuscular [IM], subcutaneous [SC])
- Topical (transdermal)—absorbed across skin or mucous membrane
- Inhalation—inhaled directly into lung to elicit local effects
- Rectal and vaginal suppository—inserted for local effects

NURSING IMPLICATIONS

1. Only administer medications you have prepared.
2. Read medication label carefully; not all formulations of parenteral medications are appropriate for IV administration (e.g., insulin for IV use).
3. Know your medications.
   - Why is this patient receiving this medication?
   - What nursing observations will tell you the desired medication action is occurring?
   - What are the nursing implications specific to this medication?
4. Do not leave medications at the bedside.
5. Check medication compatibility if administering IV.
6. Medications prepared for one route may differ in concentration for another different route (e.g., epinephrine SC is concentrated, whereas IV preparation is dilute).
   - Administering a SC epinephrine preparation IV could be fatal because of an overstimulation of the cardiac system.
7. Use at least two identifiers to determine the correct patient before administering any type of medication (e.g., armband with barcode and date of birth).
8. Have another nurse check medication calculations.
9. IM injections:
   - Do not inject more than 3 mL at one time.
   - Use the smallest gauge needle necessary to administer medication correctly

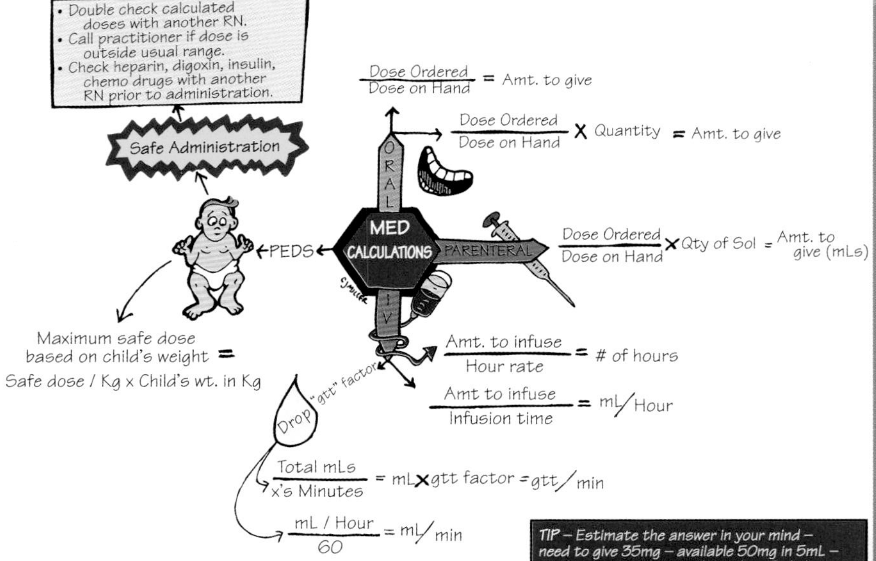

• Double check calculated doses with another RN.
• Call practitioner if dose is outside usual range.
• Check heparin, digoxin, insulin, chemo drugs with another RN prior to administration.
Safe Administration
Dose Ordered / Dose on Hand = Amt. to give
Dose Ordered / Dose on Hand X Quantity = Amt. to give
ORAL
MED CALCULATIONS
PEDS
PARENTERAL
Dose Ordered / Dose on Hand X Qty of Sol = Amt. to give (mLs)
IV
Maximum safe dose based on child's weight = Safe dose / Kg x Child's wt. in Kg
Amt. to infuse / Hour rate = # of hours
"gtt" factor
Drop
Amt to infuse / Infusion time = mL/Hour
Total mLs / x's Minutes = mL X gtt factor = gtt/min
mL / Hour / 60 = mL/min
TIP – Estimate the answer in your mind – need to give 35mg – available 50mg in 5mL – you know your answer is less than 5mL, but over 2.5 mL.
© 2016 Nursing Education Consultants, Inc.

What You Need to Know

Medication Calculation

METHODS OF CALCULATION

- Drugs requiring individualized dosing can be calculated by body weight (BW) or body surface area (BSA).
- BW and BSA methods are useful when calculating pediatric medications and antineoplastic medications, as well as for patients with low BW, patients who are obese, or older adults.
- Before calculating a dose, all units of measurement should be converted to a single system, preferably what is on the drug label. *For example:* If the medication is supplied in milligrams (mg) and the drug is ordered in grams (g), then convert the g to mg.

NURSING IMPLICATIONS

1. Always have another registered nurse (RN) double-check medications when you have to calculate the dosage.
2. Consult the health care provider if the dosage is outside the recommended range.
3. Do not administer medications if someone else has calculated the dose for you; administer only those medications you have calculated and prepared.
4. Be very cautious about calculating drug dosages for pediatric patients.
5. Even when an intravenous (IV) pump for the patient is in place, you still need to know how many milliliters per hour the IV should be infusing. This infusion rate is important to know to set the pump and to check the accuracy of delivery.
6. The West Nomogram uses a child's height and weight to determine the BSA. The BSA formula is used to determine the medication dosage for a specific pediatric patient.

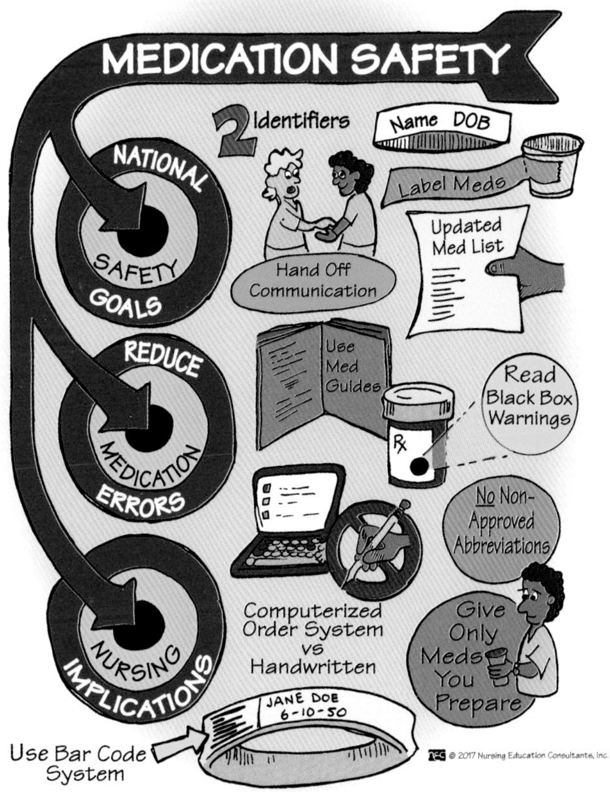
MEDICATION SAFETY
NATIONAL SAFETY GOALS
REDUCE MEDICATION ERRORS
NURSING IMPLICATIONS
2 Identifiers
Name DOB
Label Meds
Hand Off Communication
Updated Med List
Use Med Guides
Rx
Read Black Box Warnings
No Non-Approved Abbreviations
Computerized Order System vs Handwritten
Give Only Meds You Prepare
JANE DOE 6-10-50
Use Bar Code System
© 2017 Nursing Education Consultants, Inc.

What You Need to Know

Medication Safety

NATIONAL PATIENT SAFETY GOALS

- Identify patients correctly using two identifiers, such as the patient's armband and date of birth.
- Provide important test results to the right person on time.
- Before a procedure, label medications that are not labeled (e.g., medication in syringes), and do this in the area where the medication is set up.
- Use handoff communication techniques to pass along correct information about a patient's medication.
- Review new medications with current medications and be sure patient understands.
- Have patient bring an up-to-date list of medications every time there is a visit to the health care provider.

REDUCE MEDICATION ERRORS

- Use Medication Guides (MedGuides), which are approved by the U.S. Federal Drug Administration (FDA) and created to educate patients about how to minimize harm from potentially dangerous drugs.
- Review all *black box warnings* before administering medication.
- The Institute of Medicine (IOM) identifies three categories of fatal medication errors: human factors (e.g., administering a drug IV instead of IM), communication mistakes (e.g., illegible handwriting of an order), and name confusion (e.g., medications that sound like or look like another medication).

NURSING IMPLICATIONS

1. All high-alert medications should have a safety checklist.
2. Replace handwritten medication orders with a computerized order entry system (CPOE).
3. Ensure that a clinical pharmacist accompanies ICU physicians on rounds.
4. Avoid using error-prone abbreviations; see "Do Not Use List" from the Joint Commission.
5. Conduct a medication reconciliation by comparing what medications the patient is currently taking with a list of new medications being prescribed.
6. Use a computerized bar-code system that matches the patient's armband bar code to a drug bar code.
7. Administer only medications that you prepare.
8. Have two nurses sign off on high-risk medications (e.g., epinephrine, insulin,

EAR DROPS ADMINISTRATION

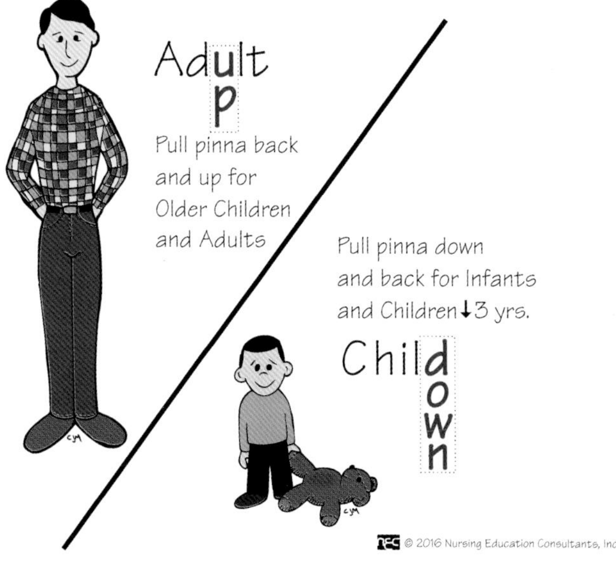

What You Need to Know

Ear Drop Administration

PROCEDURE

- Position patient supine on his or her side with affected ear up.
- Medication should be at least room temperature, not cold.
- Open ear canal of an adult by drawing back on the pinna and slightly upward.
- Open ear canal of a child less than 3 years of age by drawing back on the pinna and slightly downward.
- Allow the prescribed number of drops to fall along the inside of the ear and flow into the ear by gravity. Do not attempt to put the drops directly on the eardrum.
- Have patient remain supine for a few minutes to keep the medication from leaking out.

USES

- Treat ear infections
- Dissolve earwax (cerumen)
- Decrease pain

NURSING IMPLICATIONS

1. If medication is not instilled at room temperature, the patient may experience vertigo, dizziness, pain, and nausea.
2. If ear drainage is observed, assess patient and determine whether the eardrum is ruptured. If ruptured, do not administer medication until health care provider is consulted.
3. Do not occlude ear canal with dropper or syringe.
4. Never force medication into an occluded ear canal; doing so creates pressure, which could damage or rupture the eardrum.

Important nursing implications | Serious/life-threatening implications
Most frequent side effects | Patient teaching

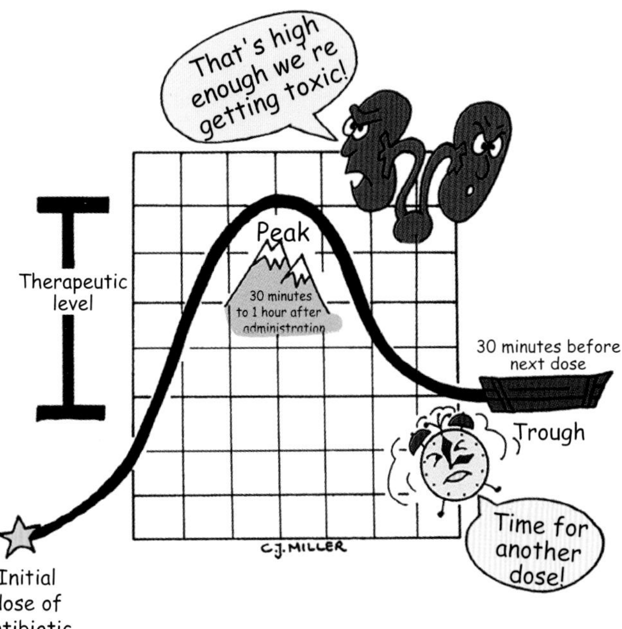
PEAK AND TROUGH
That's high enough we're getting toxic!
Therapeutic level
Peak
30 minutes to 1 hour after administration
30 minutes before next dose
Trough
Time for another dose!
Initial dose of antibiotic
C.J. MILLER

What You Need to Know

Peak and Trough

USES

- Is primarily used to monitor levels of the aminoglycoside family of antibiotics. Monitoring serum drug levels enables the physician to individualize dosage levels to maximal effectiveness, which allows drug levels to be at an effective but not toxic level.
- If the patient is on a once-daily dose, the physician will often focus on the *trough* level instead of the *peak* level. The serum level of the medication must drop down to a designated level. One daily dose means that the highest peak level is guaranteed when the daily dose is given.
- When multiple daily doses are given, both peak and trough levels must be measured. The timing of the levels drawn is important for accuracy.
- The peak level (highest blood level of drug) is usually 1 to 3 hours after oral administration. Levels are usually drawn 30 minutes to 1 hour after an intramuscular (IM) injection, 30 minutes after completion of an intravenous (IV) infusion, or at the drug's proposed peak time.
- If the patient is taking multiple doses, the trough sample (lowest blood level of drug) should be taken just before the next dose.

NURSING IMPLICATIONS

1. If the trough level is too high, toxicity can occur. Nephrotoxicity and ototoxicity are primary problems of the aminoglycosides.
2. If the peak is too low, no or minimal therapeutic effect is achieved.
3. Check laboratory values for peak and trough levels.
4. Report serum levels that are not within established ranges of peak and trough levels.
5. Explain to the patient the purpose for measurement of the peak and trough levels.
6. Maintain accuracy of values; ensure that serum laboratory values are drawn at scheduled times.
7. Risk of toxicity is increased in patients with decreased renal function.

Important nursing implications   Serious/life-threatening implications

Most frequent side effects   Patient teaching

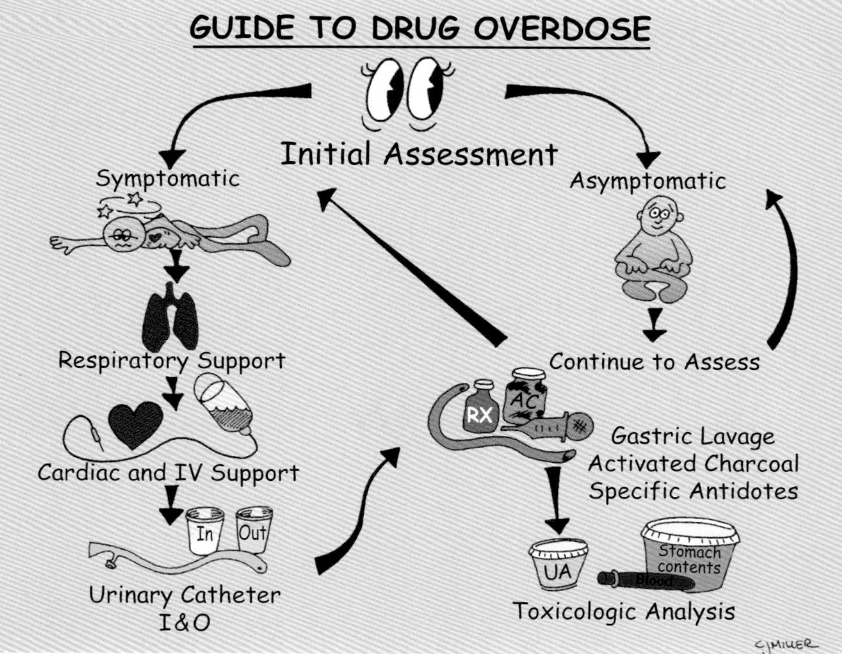
GUIDE TO DRUG OVERDOSE
Initial Assessment
Symptomatic
Asymptomatic
Respiratory Support
Continue to Assess
RX
AC
Cardiac and IV Support
Gastric Lavage
Activated Charcoal
Specific Antidotes
In
Out
UA
Stomach contents
Blood
Urinary Catheter
I&O
Toxicologic Analysis
CJMILLER

What You Need to Know

Guide to Drug Overdose

NURSING MANAGEMENT

1. Make an initial assessment, including vital signs and level of consciousness.
2. The specific drug taken in the overdose will dictate the treatment.
   - Obtain information about amount of drug, time, and underlying medical problems.
   - Direct family member or other individual to bring drug and/or container to the emergency department.
   - If depressant drug effects are present, naloxone (Narcan) and flumazenil (Romazicon) may be administered, because naloxone counteracts opiate effects and flumazenil reverses the effects of benzodiazepine overdose.
3. Perform gastric lavage to remove unabsorbed drugs mechanically from the stomach.
4. Activated charcoal may be given to help bind drugs and keep them in the stomach and intestines.
   - Activated charcoal reduces the amount of drug absorbed into the blood.
   - The drug, bound to the charcoal, is then expelled in the stool.
5. Respiratory and cardiac support may be required for symptomatic cases.
6. Intravenous lines, laboratory tests for toxicologic analysis, and a urinary catheter may also be ordered.

Helpful mnemonic for opiate overdose:

Cool to the touch and unresponsive to pain.
Hunger diminished and scars over vein.
Pupils pinpointed and blood pressure low.
Urine diminished and breathing slow.

Another mnemonic to help you remember the most rapid (speedy) way toxins or medications enter the body:

4 **S**s—**S**tick it, **S**niff it, **S**uck it, **S**oak it
Stick: injection; **S**niff: inhalation; **S**uck: ingestion; **S**oak: absorption

---

Important nursing implications | Serious/life-threatening implications
Most frequent side effects | Patient teaching

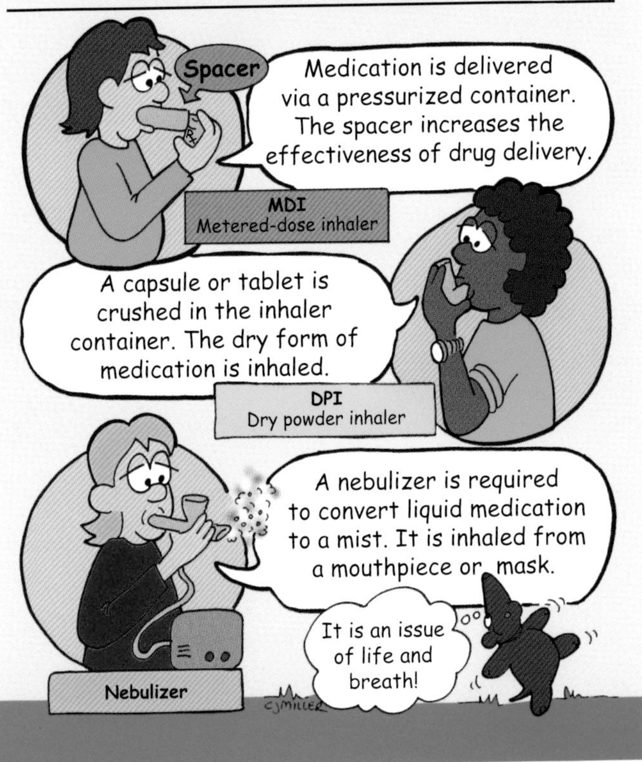
ADMINISTRATION OF MEDICATIONS BY INHALATION
Spacer
Medication is delivered via a pressurized container. The spacer increases the effectiveness of drug delivery.
MDI
Metered-dose inhaler
A capsule or tablet is crushed in the inhaler container. The dry form of medication is inhaled.
DPI
Dry powder inhaler
A nebulizer is required to convert liquid medication to a mist. It is inhaled from a mouthpiece or mask.
It is an issue of life and breath!
Nebulizer
CJMILLER

What You Need to Know

Administration of Medications by Inhalation

METERED-DOSE INHALER (MDI)

- Hand-held pressurized containers deliver a measured dose of medication with each "puff."
- Dosing may require two "puffs"—patient should wait 1 minute between "puffs."
- A spacer device may be used to increase the delivery of medication and to decrease medication deposited in mouth and throat. Pediatric patients often require the spacer.
- Requires "hand-lung coordination"—patient should exhale and, on beginning of inhalation, activate the MDI.
- Patient should hold his or her breath for approximately 10 seconds after inhalation.

DRY POWDER INHALER (DPI)

- Each medication comes with a delivery system. Medication should be administered only with delivery system provided. No aerosol propellant is used.
- Capsules and tablets are to be administered by inhalation only; medications *are not to be taken by mouth*.
- Delivery system crushes medication to a fine powder to be inhaled.
- After system is loaded, teach patient to cover mouthpiece and inhale deeply.
- Compared with MDIs, medication delivery is significantly more efficient.

SMALL-VOLUME NEBULIZERS

- A small machine converts a medication solution to a nebulized or mist form.
- Prescribed amount of medication is added to a nebulizer cup or container and attached to the machine.
- Determining whether a diluent needs to be added to the medication to facilitate the delivery is important.
- Most effective method of delivery is via mouthpiece; however, medication may also be delivered via face mask.
- When the mist begins to form at the end of mouthpiece, ask patient to seal his or her mouth over mouthpiece and start a slow, deep breath; patient should hold his or her breath for a short time and then exhale slowly.
- Mouth should be rinsed after treatment, and equipment should be rinsed and allowed to dry. Do not store wet equipment.
- With inhaled steroid medications, mouth should be rinsed to prevent infections.

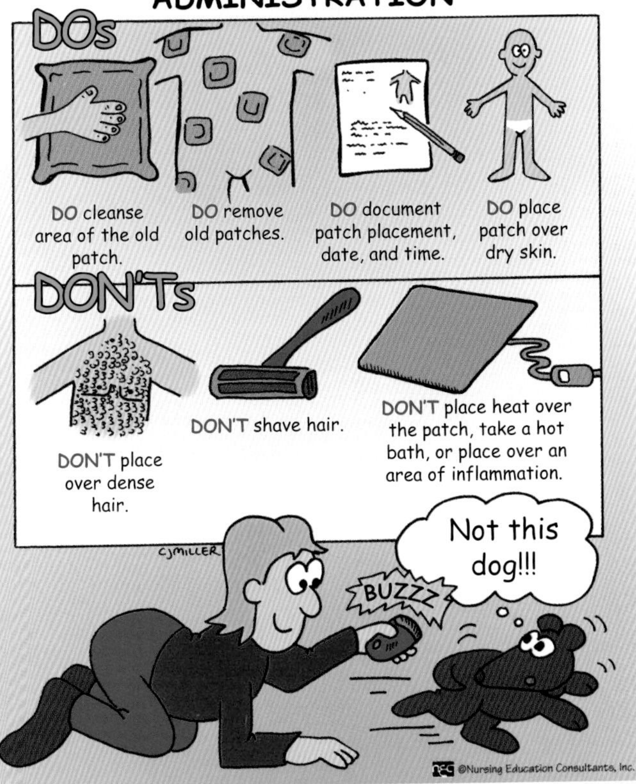
TRANSDERMAL MEDICATION ADMINISTRATION
DOs
DO cleanse area of the old patch.
DO remove old patches.
DO document patch placement, date, and time.
DO place patch over dry skin.
DON'Ts
DON'T place over dense hair.
DON'T shave hair.
DON'T place heat over the patch, take a hot bath, or place over an area of inflammation.
CJMILLER
BUZZZ
Not this dog!!!
©Nursing Education Consultants, Inc.

What You Need to Know

Transdermal Medication Administration

GENERAL

- Transdermal medications are administered topically and absorbed through the skin into the blood; they can exert a systemic effect.
- Avoids first-pass metabolism and decreases bioavailability of medication.
- Provides a controlled, constant release of medication.
- Patients who are obese or diaphoretic may have difficulty absorbing the medication.
- If a patient is going to have a magnetic resonance imaging (MRI) procedure, make sure the patch of transdermal medication does not contain a metallic component. The U.S. Food and Drug Administration (FDA) recommends that health care professionals note the presence of a patch when they refer patients for an MRI. The patch may be removed before the MRI and replaced after the exam is completed.
- Heat increases the absorption of transdermal medications. Check with the health care provider (HCP) before administering a medication patch to a patient who has a temperature higher than 102°F.
- Do not apply any heat over patch; doing so will increase absorption of medication.
- Do not allow medication to come in direct contact with fingers.

ADMINISTRATION GUIDELINES

1. Follow principles of medication administration.
2. Apply patch to dry, hairless area of subcutaneous tissue—preferably the chest, abdomen, or upper back.
3. Remove old patch and cleanse area; apply new patch in a different area.
4. Do not apply a patch over an area of emaciated skin or on an area with irritated or broken skin.
5. Do not apply an adhesive dressing over the patch.
6. Dispose old patches according to facility guidelines. Of specific concern is proper disposal of fentanyl patches.

Important nursing implications | Serious/life-threatening implications
Most frequent side effects | Patient teaching

MORPHINE SULFATE

The opium poppy is one of nature's ways of controlling pain.

Opium Poppy

Morphine Sulfate

CJMILLER

Most common drug for PCA—maintains even pain control.

I didn't know that, but I do know the route can be PO (TAB-LIQ), IV, IM, SC, rectal, epidural, or intrathecal.

Side effects:
- Decreased blood pressure
- Respiratory depression
- Urinary retention
- Constipation

What You Need to Know

MORPHINE SULFATE

Classification

Analgesic, opioid agonist ■ Black Box Alert ▲ High Alert

Actions

Interacts at a specific receptor-binding site. Agonist activity at the receptor site can result in analgesia, euphoria, depression, hallucinations, miosis, and sedation. Alters pain at the spinal cord and higher levels in the central nervous system (CNS) (Schedule II on Controlled Substances Act).

Uses

- Relieves severe pain
- Decreases anxiety, therefore decreases myocardial oxygen demands with pain from a myocardial infarction

Contraindications

- Hypersensitivity

Precautions

- Seizures, asthma, and severe respiratory depression
- Intracranial pressure and suspected head injuries; may mask the development of increased intracranial pressure (IICP)
- Hepatic and renal dysfunction; biliary tract surgery

Side Effects

- Respiratory depression, cough suppression
- Urinary retention, confusion
- Constipation, nausea and vomiting
- Orthostatic hypotension
- Tolerance and physical dependency with long-term use
- Toxicity: coma, respiratory depression, and pinpoint pupils

Nursing Implications

1. Perform strict documentation and inventory assessment of narcotic.
2. Assess pain and vital signs (especially respirations) before and after the dose; do not administer if respirations are less than 12 breaths per minute.
3. Infants and older adults are very sensitive to depression of respirations.
4. Naloxone (Narcan) reverses the effect of morphine.
5. Medication of choice for patient-controlled analgesia (PCA).
6. Cancer patients should receive opioids on a fixed schedule; tolerance may occur, requiring dosage escalation.

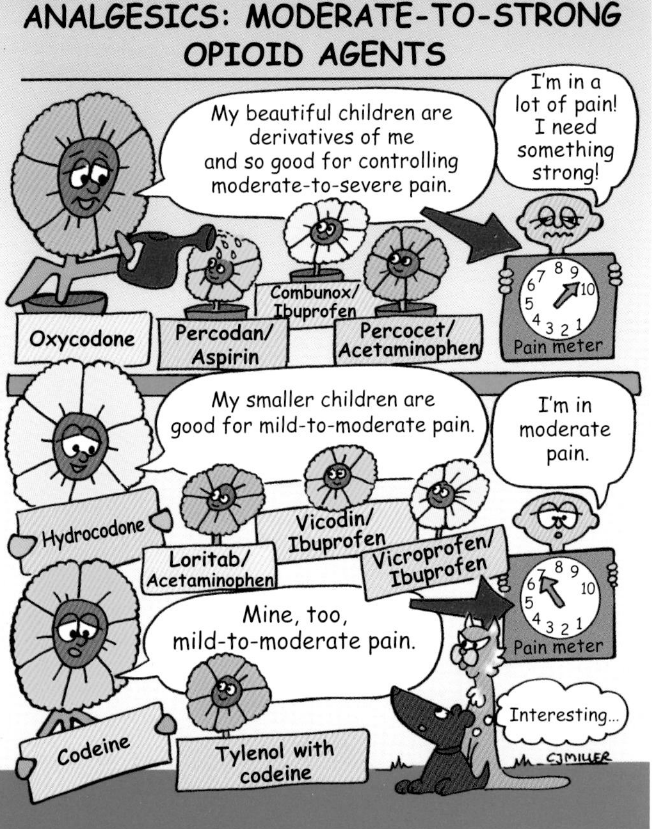
ANALGESICS: MODERATE-TO-STRONG OPIOID AGENTS
My beautiful children are derivatives of me and so good for controlling moderate-to-severe pain.
I'm in a lot of pain! I need something strong!
Oxycodone
Percodan/ Aspirin
Combunox/ Ibuprofen
Percocet/ Acetaminophen
Pain meter
My smaller children are good for mild-to-moderate pain.
I'm in moderate pain.
Hydrocodone
Loritab/ Acetaminophen
Vicodin/ Ibuprofen
Vicroprofen/ Ibuprofen
Pain meter
Mine, too, mild-to-moderate pain.
Interesting...
Codeine
Tylenol with codeine
CJMILLER

What You Need to Know

ANALGESICS: MODERATE-TO-STRONG OPIOID AGENTS

Actions

Bind with receptors in the brain and spinal cord that are associated with pain. Moderate opioid analgesics are similar to morphine; however, pain control is less effective, and the potential for respiratory depression is less.

OPIOID ANALGESICS

Oxycodone—PO Schedule II

- **Percodan**—combined with aspirin
- **Percocet**—combined with acetaminophen
- **Combunox**—combined with ibuprofen
- **OxyContin**—controlled release, dosing is usually every 12 hours with another analgesic for breakthrough pain

Hydrocodone—PO Schedule II

- **Lortab**—combined with acetaminophen
- **Vicodin**—combined with acetaminophen
- **Vicoprofen**—combined with ibuprofen
- May also be combined with antihistamines and nasal decongestants for cough suppression

Codeine—PO, IV, IM, SC Schedule II

- Tylenol with codeine (PO) for mild pain relief
- Frequently combined with various agents for suppression of cough

Nursing Implications

1. Assessment is critical to effective pain control. Carefully assess patient's level of pain and administer analgesic as ordered.
2. Follow institution procedure for administering an opioid (Controlled Substance Act).
3. Reassess patient 1 hour after administering medication.
4. Administer medication before pain returns; fixed schedule of dosing may be more efficient than "as needed" dosing.
5. Developing physical dependence is extremely rare for hospitalized patients who receive short-term therapy for pain. Even when physical dependence does occur, patients rarely develop addictive behavior; the majority go through a gradual withdrawal and never take opioids again.

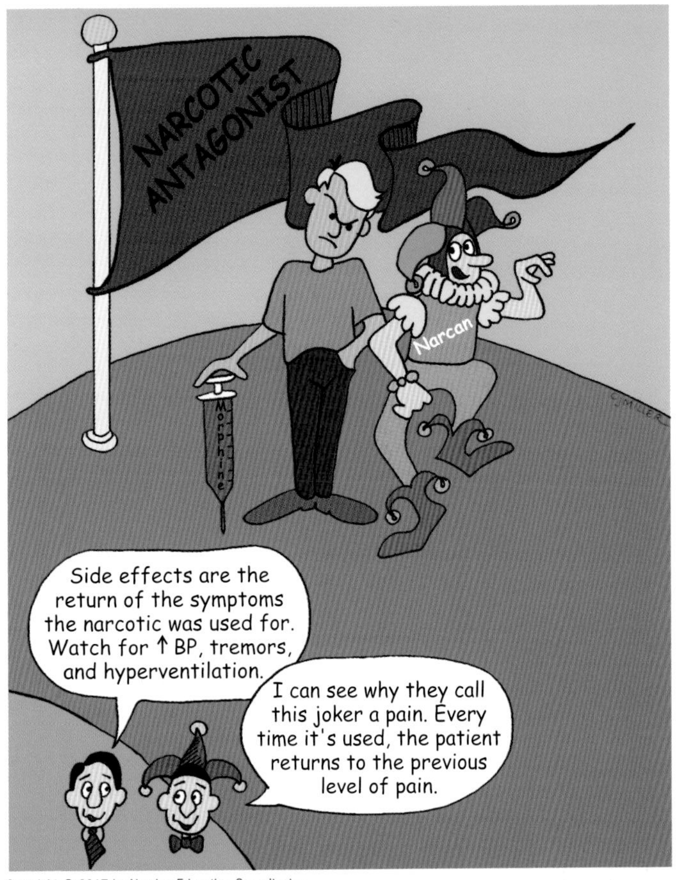
NARCOTIC ANTAGONIST
Narcan
Morphine
Side effects are the return of the symptoms the narcotic was used for. Watch for ↑ BP, tremors, and hyperventilation.
I can see why they call this joker a pain. Every time it's used, the patient returns to the previous level of pain.

What You Need to Know

NARCOTIC ANTAGONISTS: NALOXONE (NARCAN)

Actions

Opioid antagonists block (or antagonize) opiate-receptor sites. Principal use is the treatment of opioid overdose.

Uses

- Reverse the opiate effects of narcotic overdose and respiratory depression

Contraindications and Precautions

- Patients who are using nonopioid drugs
- Neonates and children
- Patients with a history of dependency; may precipitate acute withdrawal

Side Effects

- Too rapid reversal of narcotic depression—nausea, vomiting, tremors, hypertension
- Minimal pharmacologic effects in absence of narcotics
- Reversal of analgesia

Nursing Implications

1. Preferred route of administration is intravenously; response is within 1 to 2 minutes, and peak action is within 20 to 60 minutes.
2. Patient should be frequently assessed; if the narcotic analgesic lasts longer in the system than the action of the Narcan antagonist, then respiratory depression may recur.
3. If patient has a history of opioid dependency, administration of Narcan may produce symptoms of acute withdrawal.
4. If accidental poisoning or possible narcotic overdose is a concern, Narcan is usually administered.
5. Not effective against barbiturates or other central nervous system depressant medications.

Important nursing implications | Serious/life-threatening implications

Most frequent side effects | Patient teaching

So...WITH NEW PURPOSE AND STRENGTH SHE BECAME...
ASPIRIN
ASPIRIN WOMAN!

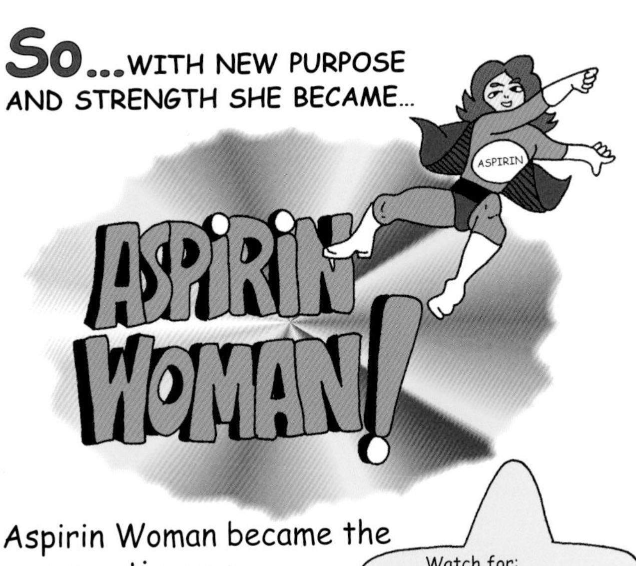

Aspirin Woman became the new antipower...

Antiinflammatory
Antipain (mild to moderate)
Antipyretic
Antiplatelet aggregation

Watch for:

- Bleeding tendencies
- Tinnitus
- Stomach pain
- Renal impairment

CJMILLER

What You Need to Know

ACETYLSALICYLIC ACID (ASA)—ASPIRIN

Classification

Analgesic, antipyretic, antiplatelet; nonsteroidal antiinflammatory drug (first-generation NSAID) ▲ High Alert

Action

Is a nonselective cyclooxygenase inhibitor that decreases the formation of prostaglandins involved in the production of inflammation, pain, and fever. Inhibits platelet aggregation.

Uses

- Relieves low-to-moderate pain
- Decreases inflammation in systemic lupus erythematosus, rheumatoid arthritis, osteoarthritis, bursitis, and tendonitis
- Is a prophylactic medication to reduce the risk of transient ischemic attack, ischemic stroke, and myocardial infarction

Contraindications and Precautions

- Hypersensitivity to salicylates
- Do not use during pregnancy
- History of gastrointestinal (GI) ulceration, peptic ulcer disease (PUD), or any bleeding disorder
- Use in children with a recent history of viral infection (e.g., influenza, chickenpox) has been associated with Reye syndrome

Side Effects

- Decreases platelet aggregation; increases bleeding potential
- Epigastric distress, heartburn, and nausea
- Aspirin overdose or toxicity—respiratory alkalosis that progresses to respiratory depression and acidosis; hyperthermia, sweating, and dehydration with electrolyte imbalance; tinnitus, headache

Nursing Implications

1. Give with milk or full glass of water to decrease gastric irritation.
2. Teach safety measures to parents regarding medications at home.
3. The potential for toxicity is high in older adults and children.
4. Teach patient to avoid concurrent use of alcohol to decrease GI irritation.
5. Patient should not take aspirin for at least 1 week before surgery.
6. Evaluate patient to determine purpose of medication—pain, inflammation, or antiplatelet action.

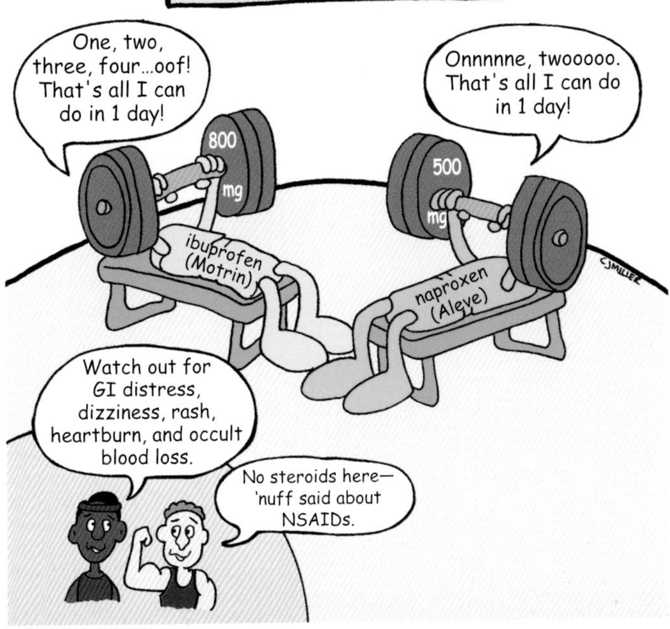
NSAID GYM
NO PAIN, NO FLAME, AND NO HEAT WHEN WE MEET
(ANALGESIC, ANTIINFLAMMATORY, ANTIPYRETIC)
One, two, three, four...oof! That's all I can do in 1 day!
Onnnnne, twooooo. That's all I can do in 1 day!
800 mg
ibuprofen (Motrin)
500 mg
naproxen (Aleve)
CJMILLER
Watch out for GI distress, dizziness, rash, heartburn, and occult blood loss.
No steroids here—'nuff said about NSAIDs.

What You Need to Know

FIRST-GENERATION NONSTEROIDAL ANTIINFLAMMATORY DRUGS (NSAIDs)—NONASPIRIN

Actions

Suppress inflammation by inhibiting both cyclooxygenases 1 and 2 (COX-1 and COX-2), enzymes that are responsible for the synthesis of prostaglandins. NSAIDs inhibit the formation and release of prostaglandin.

Examples of First-Generation NSAIDs

Ibuprofen (e.g., Motrin, Advil, Nuprin), naproxen (Aleve), indomethacin (Indocin), piroxicam (Feldene), sulindac (Clinoril), and numerous others

Uses

- Primary use is for rheumatoid arthritis and osteoarthritis
- Reduce inflammation, pain of dysmenorrhea, and headache
- Decrease fever

CONTRAINDICATIONS AND PRECAUTIONS

- History of gastrointestinal (GI) inflammation, ulceration, and bleeding are present.
- Is not recommended for use during pregnancy.
- Do not take before or immediately after coronary artery bypass graft (CABG) surgery.
- Can cause increased risk of renal insufficiency in older patients with other chronic conditions.

Side Effects

- Dyspepsia, anorexia, nausea, vomiting, fluid retention
- Rash, dizziness, heartburn, GI bleeding

Nursing Implications

1. Take with food or milk to reduce GI distress.
2. Instruct patient to use correct concentrations for age group (e.g., infants, children).
3. Do not crush or chew enteric-coated tablets.
4. Teach patient to avoid alcohol and aspirin products while taking NSAIDs.
5. Patient should avoid all NSAIDs for a least 1 week before surgery or invasive diagnostics.
6. Nonaspirin NSAIDs do not protect against myocardial infarction (MI) and stroke, like aspirin does; in fact, they increase the risk of thrombotic events with risk being the highest with indomethacin (Indocin), sulindac (Clinoril), and meloxicam (Mobic).

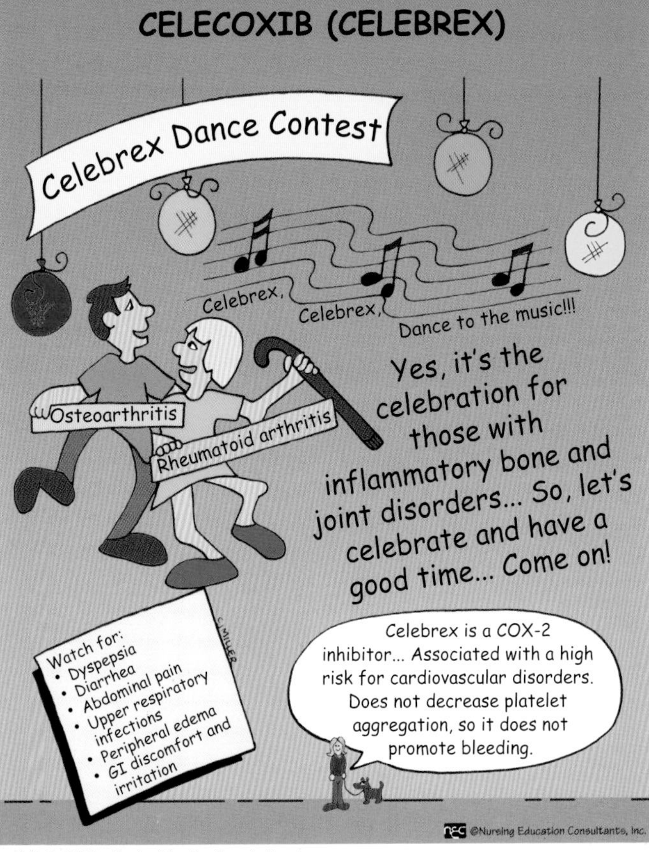
CELECOXIB (CELEBREX)
Celebrex Dance Contest
Celebrex,
Celebrex,
Dance to the music!!!
Yes, it's the celebration for those with inflammatory bone and joint disorders... So, let's celebrate and have a good time... Come on!
Osteoarthritis
Rheumatoid arthritis
Watch for:
• Dyspepsia
• Diarrhea
• Abdominal pain
• Upper respiratory infections
• Peripheral edema
• GI discomfort and irritation
C.J. MILLER
Celebrex is a COX-2 inhibitor... Associated with a high risk for cardiovascular disorders. Does not decrease platelet aggregation, so it does not promote bleeding.
©Nursing Education Consultants, Inc.

What You Need to Know

SECOND-GENERATION NSAIDs (COX-2 INHIBITOR, COXIB: CELEBREX)

Classification

Analgesic, antiinflammatory; nonsteroidal antiinflammatory drug (NSAID)

Action

Inhibits prostaglandin synthesis by selectively inhibiting cyclooxygenase 2 (COX-2), an enzyme needed for biosynthesis, which suppresses pain and inflammation while posing a lower risk of gastric ulceration

Uses

- Relieves low-to-moderate pain
- Decreases inflammation in systemic lupus erythematosus, rheumatoid arthritis, osteoarthritis

Contraindications and Precautions

- May increase the risk of myocardial infarction (MI) and stroke and other serious cardiovascular events.
- Do not use during pregnancy, especially the third trimester.
- Can impair renal function.
- Can precipitate an allergic reaction in patients allergic to sulfonamides.
- Do not use in patients with a history of hypertension, edema, heart failure, or kidney disease.

Side Effects

- Dyspepsia, abdominal pain, fatigue, nervousness, paresthesia
- Does not decrease platelet aggregation; hence, does not promote bleeding

Nursing Implications

1. Give with milk or full glass of water to enhance absorption.
2. Do not break, crush, chew, or dissolve caps. Caps can be opened into applesauce or soft food, but must be ingested immediately with water.
3. Teach patient to avoid concurrent use of alcohol to decrease gastrointestinal (GI) irritation.
4. Monitor for GI irritation, bleeding episodes, or renal impairment.
5. Evaluate patient to determine purpose of medication—reduction in pain and inflammation.
6. Teach patient to avoid use of NSAIDs to prevent vaccination-associated fever and pain, as they may blunt the immune response to the vaccine.

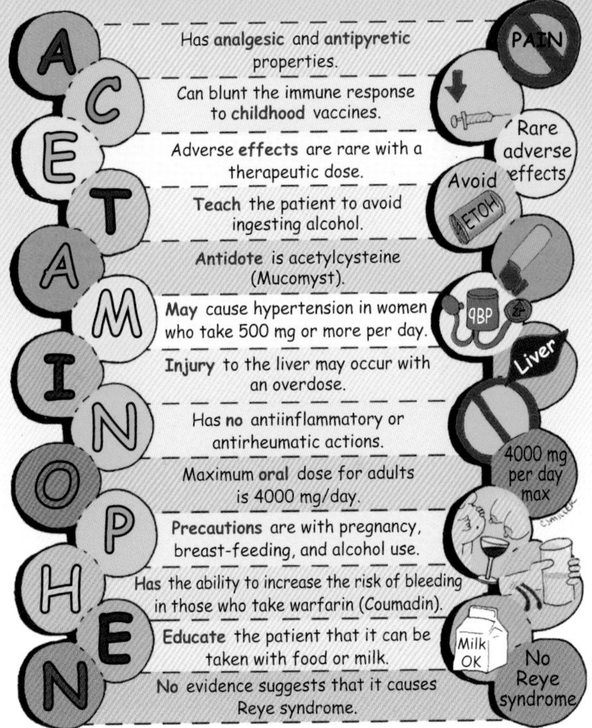
ACETAMINOPHEN
A C E T A M I N O P H E N
Has analgesic and antipyretic properties.
Can blunt the immune response to childhood vaccines.
Adverse effects are rare with a therapeutic dose.
Teach the patient to avoid ingesting alcohol.
Antidote is acetylcysteine (Mucomyst).
May cause hypertension in women who take 500 mg or more per day.
Injury to the liver may occur with an overdose.
Has no antiinflammatory or antirheumatic actions.
Maximum oral dose for adults is 4000 mg/day.
Precautions are with pregnancy, breast-feeding, and alcohol use.
Has the ability to increase the risk of bleeding in those who take warfarin (Coumadin).
Educate the patient that it can be taken with food or milk.
No evidence suggests that it causes Reye syndrome.
PAIN
Rare adverse effects
Avoid
ETOH
BP
Liver
4000 mg per day max
Milk OK
No Reye syndrome
©Nursing Education Consultants, Inc.

What You Need to Know

ACETAMINOPHEN (TYLENOL)

Classification

Analgesic, antipyretic

Action

Decreases prostaglandin synthesis in the CNS and has antipyretic and analgesic action. Does not possess antiinflammatory properties, does not cause gastric ulceration, does not suppress platelet aggregation or impair renal blood flow or function.

Uses

- Relieves low-to-moderate pain, fever
- Arthralgia, dental pain, dysmenorrhea, headache
- Preferred drug for children having chickenpox or influenza (not associated with Reye syndrome)

Contraindications and Precautions

- Hypersensitivity
- Precaution during pregnancy and breast-feeding
- Excessive alcohol ingestion

Side Effects

- Adverse effects rare at therapeutic doses
- Overdose or toxicity leads to liver damage

Nursing Implications

1. Give with milk or full glass of water to decrease gastric irritation.
2. Teach parents that drug may blunt the immune response to childhood vaccines and should not be given to treat pain or fever associated with the vaccination.
3. Teach patient to avoid concurrent use of alcohol to prevent liver damage.
4. Evaluate patient to determine purpose of medication—pain or fever.
5. Antidote for overdose is acetylcysteine (Mucomyst).
6. If patient is taking warfarin (Coumadin), concurrent use of acetaminophen has ability to increase risk of bleeding.
7. Monitor medications that may contain acetaminophen, so as not to exceed maximum recommended dose.

Important nursing implications | Serious/life-threatening implications

Most frequent side effects | Patient teaching

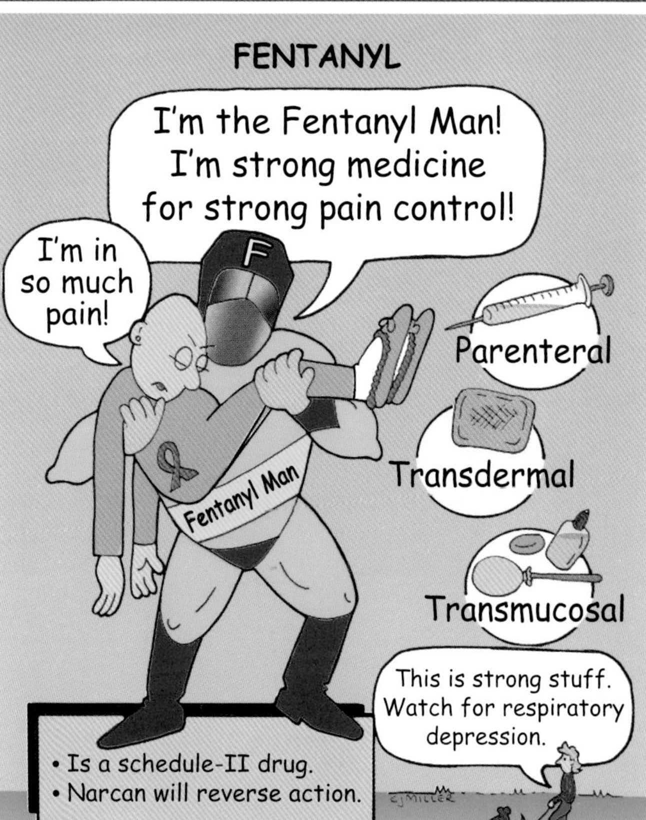
FENTANYL
I'm the Fentanyl Man! I'm strong medicine for strong pain control!
I'm in so much pain!
F
Fentanyl Man
Parenteral
Transdermal
Transmucosal
This is strong stuff. Watch for respiratory depression.
• Is a schedule-II drug.
• Narcan will reverse action.
©Nursing Education Consultants, Inc.

What You Need to Know

FENTANYL

Classification

Strong narcotic analgesic; Schedule II of Controlled Substances Act

Uses

- Fentanyl (IM, IV)—facilitates the induction of anesthesia; may be used with droperidol
- Transdermal (Duragesic patches)—relief of persistent pain is reported in patients who are tolerant of opioid agents
- Transmucosal (lozenge on a stick [Actiq]; buccal film [Onsolis]; buccal tablets [Fentora]; sublingual tablets [Abstral]; sublingual spray [Subsys]; transnasal spray [Lazanda])—breakthrough pain in patients with cancer who are opioid tolerant

Contraindications

- Is only indicated for the relief of severe pain.
- In patients with suspected head injuries, fentanyl may mask the development of increased intracranial pressure (IICP).

Side Effects

- Respiratory depression
- Sedation, euphoria, and constipation
- Hypotension, pupillary miosis, urinary retention, nausea
- Tolerance and physical dependency with long-term use

Nursing Implications

1. Perform strict documentation and inventory assessment of narcotic.
2. Assess pain and vital signs (especially respirations) before and after the dose; do not administer if respirations are less than 12 breaths per minute.
3. Pay close attention to guidelines for administration.
4. Patch is used for opioid-tolerant patients, not for control of postoperative pain.
5. Respiratory depression can be reversed with naloxone (Narcan).
6. Teach patients to avoid exposing the patch to external heat sources (e.g., heating pads, hot baths, electric blankets); doing so can accelerate the release of the medication, as can fever, sunbathing, and strenuous exercise.
7. Teach client that if intranasal spray has not been used within 5 days, the bottle should be reprimed by spraying once and/or discarded and replaced with a new one.

Important nursing implications | Serious/life-threatening implications

Most frequent side effects | Patient teaching

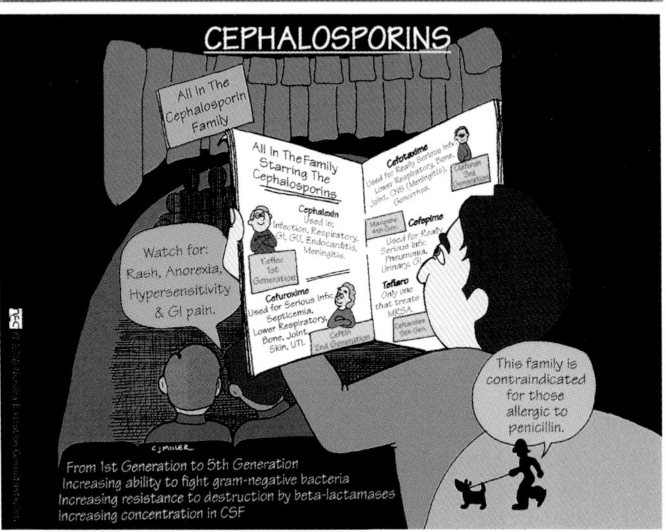
CEPHALOSPORINS
All In The Cephalosporin Family
All In The Family Starring The Cephalosporins
Cephalexin
Used In: Infection, Respiratory, GI, GU, Endocarditis, Meningitis.
Keflex 1st Generation
Cefuroxime
Used for Serious Infc Septicemia, Lower Respiratory, Bone, Joint, Skin, UTI.
Ceftin 2nd Generation
Cefotaxime
Used for Really Serious Infc. Lower Respiratory, Bone, Joint, CNS (Meningitis), Gonorrhea.
Claforan 3rd Generation
Maxipime 4th Gen.
Cefepime
Used for Really Serious Infc Pneumonia, Urinary, GI
Teflaro
Only one that treats MRSA.
Ceftaroline 5th Gen.
Watch for: Rash, Anorexia, Hypersensitivity & GI pain.
This family is contraindicated for those allergic to penicillin.
CJ MILLER
From 1st Generation to 5th Generation
Increasing ability to fight gram-negative bacteria
Increasing resistance to destruction by beta-lactamases
Increasing concentration in CSF

What You Need to Know

CEPHALOSPORINS

Action

Each generation has increasing bactericidal activity to break down gram-negative bacteria and anaerobes, as well as to reach the cerebrospinal fluid. Cephalosporins interfere with bacterial cell wall synthesis and are considered broad-spectrum. The cell weakens, swells, bursts, and dies as a result of increased osmotic pressure inside the cell. Increased cephalosporin resistance is caused by production of beta-lactamases.

Uses

Gram-negative and gram-positive bacterial infections; is not active against viral or fungal infections

Caution

Do not use in patients with a severe penicillin allergy (anaphylaxis, hives).

Side Effects (Very Similar to Penicillin)

- Hypersensitivity reactions: rash, pruritus, fever.
- Anorexia, nausea, flatulence, vomiting, diarrhea.
- Can promote a *Clostridium difficile* infection.
- Severe immediate anaphylactic reactions are rare.
- Ceftriaxone and cefotetan may cause bleeding tendencies.
- Taking cefotetan or cefazolin and drinking alcohol may cause a serious disulfiram-like reaction.

Nursing Implications

1. Evaluate intramuscular (IM) and intravenous (IV) sites for reaction, such as abscess and thrombophlebitis. Minimize complication of thrombophlebitis by rotating injection sites and slowly injecting in a dilute solution.
2. IM injections are frequently painful; forewarn patient.
3. Do not reconstitute ceftriaxone with any calcium diluents (Ringer solution).
4. Notify health care provider (HCP) if diarrhea occurs—can promote development of *Clostridium difficile* infection.
5. Monitor renal and hepatic studies throughout therapy.
6. With medications that cause bleeding tendencies, monitor for bleeding.
7. If GI upset occurs, patient can take medication with food.
8. Teach patient to refrigerate oral suspensions.
9. Instruct patient to report any signs of allergy (e.g., skin rash, itching, hives).

TETRACYCLINE USES

Chlamydia, Lyme Disease,
Pneumonia (*Mycoplasma pneumoniae*)
Rocky Mountain Spotted Fever
Benefit Raffle
50th Annual Bikers Rally
GRAND PRIZE: A Tetracycline

Did you know tetracycline could be used to treat acne, too?
I'm zitting.
BROAD
SPECTRUM

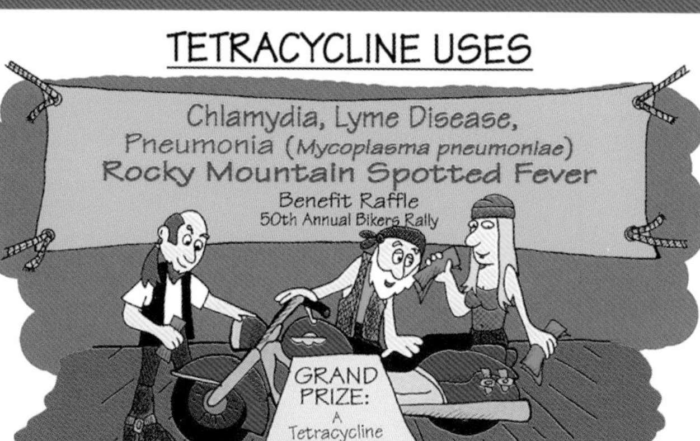

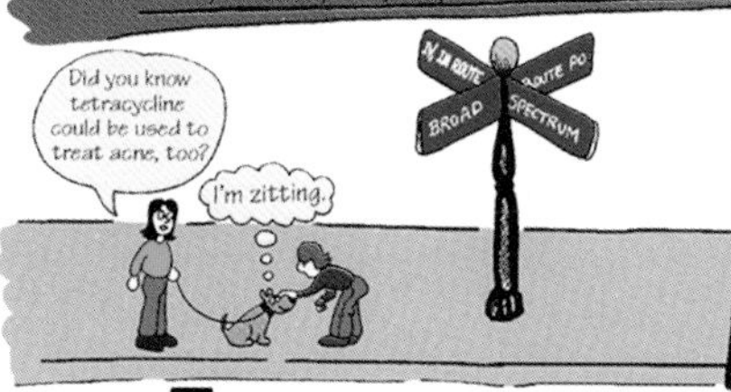

Caution:

- Staining of deciduous teeth if taken after 4th month of pregnancy.
- Staining of permanent teeth if taken from ages 4 months to 8 years.
- Don't give with milk, calcium supplements, or antacids.

What You Need to Know

TETRACYCLINES

Classification

Antibiotics

Action

Tetracyclines are bacteriostatic, broad-spectrum antibiotics that suppress bacterial growth by inhibiting protein synthesis. Inhibit growth of both gram-negative and gram-positive bacteria.

Uses

- Rickettsial diseases (Rocky Mountain spotted fever, typhus, Q fever)
- Chlamydia infections, peptic ulcer disease (*Helicobacter pylori* infection)
- Acne, *Mycoplasma pneumoniae,* Lyme disease, periodontal disease
- Brucellosis, cholera, anthrax

Precautions

- May exacerbate kidney impairment.
- Do not give to children younger than age 8 years or pregnant women.
- May cause staining of developing teeth.

Side Effects

- Alteration of vaginal and intestinal flora resulting in diarrhea and GI upset
- Photosensitivity, superinfection *(Clostridium difficile)*

Nursing Implications

1. Monitor carefully for diarrhea; it may indicate a superinfection of bowel (*Clostridium difficile or Staphylococci*).
2. Check dose and rate when delivering intravenously.
3. Take on an empty stomach; antacids, milk products, and iron supplements should not be consumed until at least 2 hours after dose was taken.
4. To avoid discoloration of permanent teeth, do not administer to pregnant women or children younger than age 8 years.
5. Use a straw with liquid preparations.
6. Wear sunscreen and protective clothing.

Important nursing implications | Serious/life-threatening implications

Most frequent side effects | Patient teaching

METRONIDAZOLE (FLAGYL)

Watch for:
• Nausea
• Diarrhea
• Stomatitis
• Headache
• Dry Mouth
• Fatigue
Metronidazole
(Flagyl)
Entamoeba histolytica
Giardia lamblia
Trichomoniasis
Gardnerella
H. pylori
Amebiasis
No alcohol products; may cause disulfiram-type reaction.
When they say no alcohol products, include no mouthwash, aftershave, deodorant, & bath splashes.
Wow, people are hard to figure.
© 2016 Nursing Education Consultants, Inc.

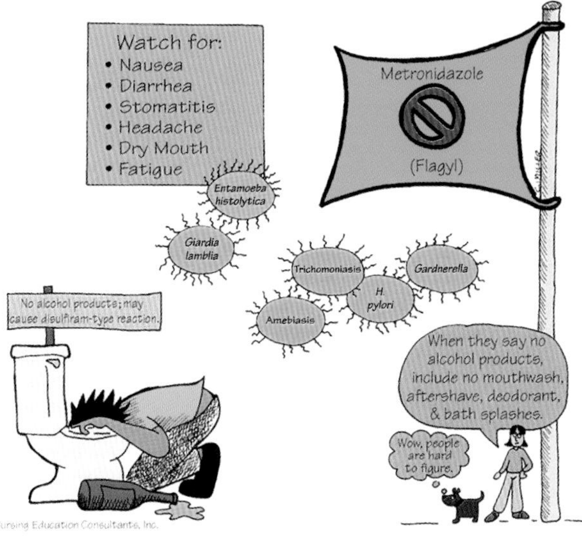

What You Need to Know

METRONIDAZOLE (FLAGYL)

Classification

Antibacterial

Action

Bacteriocidal effects against anaerobic bacterial pathogens as well as several protozoa. Interacts with cell DNA to cause strand breakage and loss of helical structure. The impairment of the DNA is responsible for the antimicrobial and mutagenic actions of the medication.

Uses

- Asymptomatic and symptomatic trichomoniasis in female and male patients
- Acute intestinal amebiasis, giardiasis, *Clostridium difficile,* and antibiotic-associated colitis
- Used in combination with tetracycline and bismuth subsalicylate (Pepto-Bismol) for treatment of *Helicobacter pylori*

Precautions

- Active central nervous system (CNS) disease, blood dyscrasias
- Avoid during first-trimester pregnancy, breast-feeding mothers
- Second- and third-trimester pregnancies, use with caution
- Alcoholism, hepatic disease

Side Effects

- Nausea, headache, dry mouth, vomiting, diarrhea, vertigo, weakness
- Metallic taste, darkening of the urine, stomatitis, insomnia
- Rarely, seizures, peripheral neuropathy, encephalopathy, aseptic meningitis

Nursing Implications

1. Take on an empty stomach if possible; may take with food if nauseated.
2. Do not use products containing alcohol (cologne, aftershave lotion, or bath splashes) or ingest alcohol products to avoid a disulfiram-type reaction (e.g., flushing, nausea and vomiting, palpitations, tachycardia, psychosis).
3. Mothers should wait until 24 hours after last dose of drug to resume breast-feeding.
4. Teach patient that harmless darkening of the urine may occur.

Important nursing implications | Serious/life-threatening implications

Most frequent side effects | Patient teaching

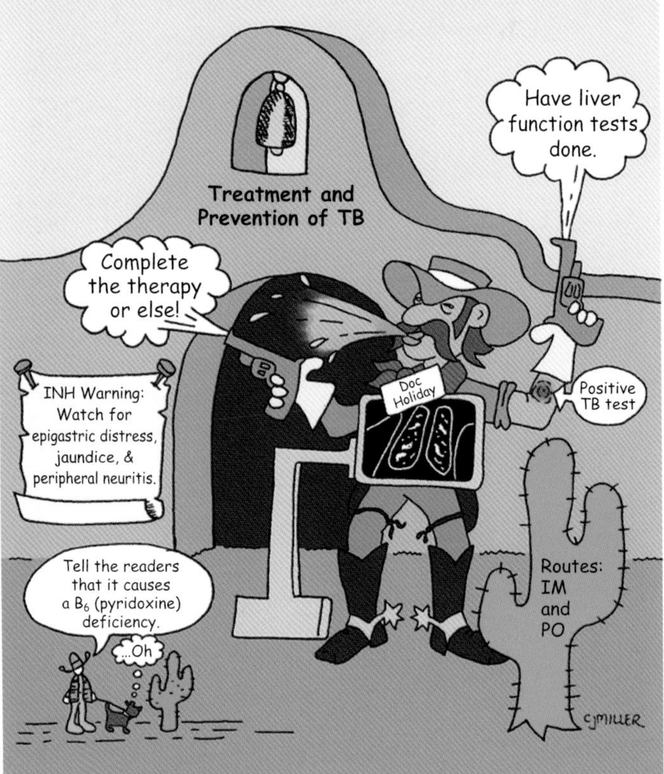
ISONIAZID (INH)
Treatment and Prevention of TB
Have liver function tests done.
Complete the therapy or else!
Doc Holiday
INH Warning: Watch for epigastric distress, jaundice, & peripheral neuritis.
Positive TB test
Tell the readers that it causes a B_6 (pyridoxine) deficiency.
...Oh
Routes: IM and PO
CJMILLER

What You Need to Know

ISONIAZID (INH)

Classification

Antimycobacterial, antituberculosis agent

Actions

Bacteriostatic to “resting organisms” and bactericidal to actively dividing organisms. Interferes with biosynthesis of bacterial protein, nucleic acid, and lipids.

Uses

- Treatment of active and latent tuberculosis
- Preventive in high-risk persons (e.g., those with a positive tuberculosis [TB] skin test or exposure)

Contraindications and Precautions

- History of isoniazid-associated hypersensitivity reaction.
- Alcoholics and patients with preexisting liver problems.
- When used to treat active TB, it must be used with another antitubercular agent.

Side Effects

- Dose-related peripheral neuropathy, clumsiness, unsteadiness, muscle ache
- Epigastric distress, jaundice, drug-induced hepatitis

Nursing Implications

1. Teach patient to take orally on an empty stomach 1 hour before or 2 hours after meals.
2. Depletes vitamin B_6 (pyridoxine) and will need supplementation during treatment.
3. Peripheral neuritis, the most common adverse effect, is preceded by paresthesias (e.g., numbness, tingling, burning, pain) of the feet and hands.
4. Teach patients to reduce or eliminate consumption of alcohol to reduce risk of hepatotoxicity.
5. Antituberculosis treatment always involves two or more medications; INH is often combined with rifampin.

Remember this mnemonic for antibiotics used in TB: **STRIPE**

ST—**st**reptomycin **R**—**r**ifampin **I**—**i**soniazid **P**—**p**yrazinamide **E**—**e**thambutol

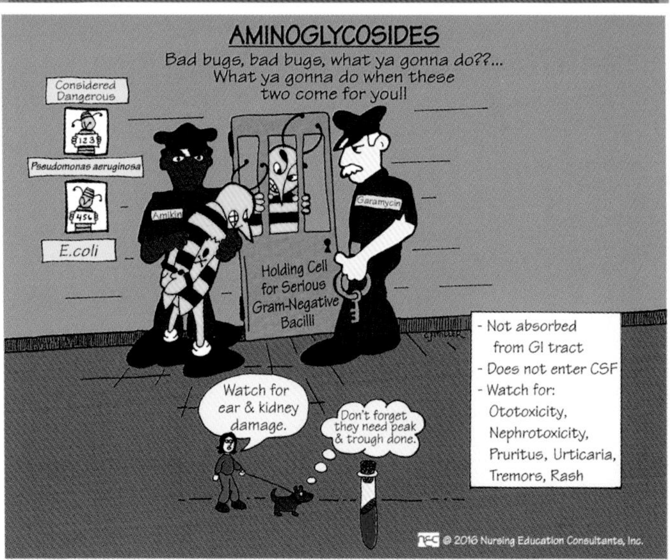
AMINOGLYCOSIDES
Bad bugs, bad bugs, what ya gonna do??...
What ya gonna do when these
two come for you!!
Considered
Dangerous
123
Pseudomonas aeruginosa
456
E.coli
Amikin
Garamycin
Holding Cell
for Serious
Gram-Negative
Bacilli
- Not absorbed
from GI tract
- Does not enter CSF
- Watch for:
Ototoxicity,
Nephrotoxicity,
Pruritus, Urticaria,
Tremors, Rash
Watch for
ear & kidney
damage.
Don't forget
they need peak
& trough done.
© 2016 Nursing Education Consultants, Inc.

What You Need to Know

AMINOGLYCOSIDES

Action

Narrow-spectrum antibiotics that are primarily effective against aerobic gram-negative bacteria. Disrupts the cell synthesis of protein; cell kill is dependent on the concentration of the medication.

Uses

- Parenteral use (poorly absorbed orally) for treatment of serious infections of the gastrointestinal, respiratory, and urinary tracts; central nervous system (CNS); bone; skin and soft tissue, including burns
- Topically for application to eyes, ears, and skin

Contraindication

- History of hypersensitivity or toxic reaction with aminoglycoside antibiotics

Precautions

- Patients who have renal impairment
- History of eighth cranial nerve impairment
- Patients with myasthenia gravis
- Possible fetal damage when given to pregnant and lactating women

Side Effects

- Nephrotoxicity (reversible injury) and ototoxicity (irreversible injury)
- Neuromuscular blockade leading to flaccid paralysis and fatal respiratory depression; increased risk in patients receiving skeletal muscle relaxants
- Hypersensitivity reactions: rash, urticaria, pruritus

Nursing Implications

1. Peak and trough levels should be assessed. Ototoxicity is associated with persistent high trough levels, rather than high peak levels.
2. Monitor renal function (e.g., blood urea nitrogen, creatinine levels).
3. Monitor for sensory problems (e.g., loss of hearing).
4. Instruct patients to report tinnitus, high-frequency hearing loss, persistent headache, nausea, dizziness, vertigo.
5. Anticipate antidote of IV calcium gluconate for treatment of neuromuscular blockade.

Important nursing implications | Serious/life-threatening implications

Most frequent side effects | Patient teaching

AMINOGLYCOSIDE TOXICITY

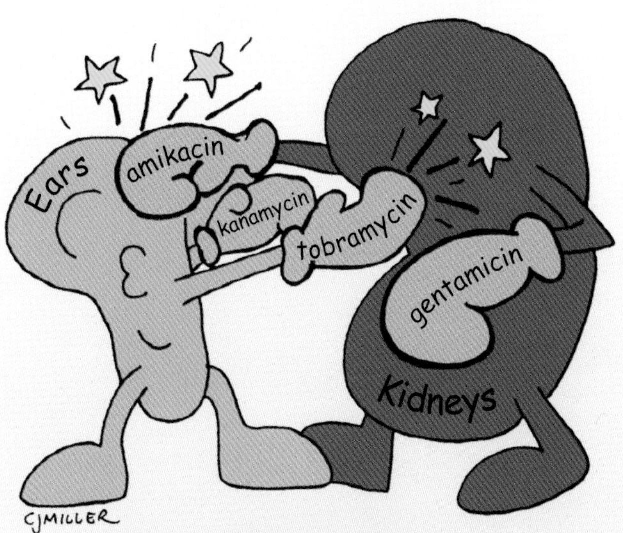

Major toxic effects of aminoglycosides are ototoxicity and nephrotoxicity.

What You Need to Know

AMINOGLYCOSIDE TOXICITY

Action (Aminoglycoside Antibiotics)

Bactericidal against gram-negative bacteria (narrow-spectrum) and certain gram-positive organisms. Disrupts bacterial protein synthesis. Is used for serious infections.

Contraindications and Precautions

- History of hypersensitivity or toxic reaction with aminoglycoside antibiotics
- Patients with renal impairment, history of eighth cranial nerve impairment
- Patients with myasthenia gravis
- Neonates

Toxicity

- Nephrotoxicity (reversible injury) and ototoxicity (irreversible injury).
- Neuromuscular blockade can lead to flaccid paralysis, and fatal respiratory depression can occur in patients receiving skeletal muscle relaxants.

Drug Interactions

- Ethacrynic acid (Edecrin) significantly increases ototoxicity.
- Amphotericin B, cephalosporins, polymyxins, vancomycin, cyclosporine, acetylsalicylic acid (ASA), and nonsteroidal antiinflammatory drugs (NSAIDs) increase risk of nephrotoxicity.
- Skeletal muscle relaxants and neuromuscular-blocking agents used in surgery increase risk of neuromuscular blockade.

Nursing Implications

1. Peak and trough levels should be assessed. Ototoxicity is associated with persistent high trough levels rather than high peak levels.
2. Monitor renal function (e.g., blood urea nitrogen, creatinine levels).
3. Monitor for sensory problems (e.g., loss of hearing).
4. Instruct patients to report tinnitus, high-frequency hearing loss, persistent headache, nausea, dizziness, vertigo.
5. Anticipate antidote of intravenous (IV) calcium gluconate for treatment of neuromuscular blockade.

Important nursing implications | Serious/life-threatening implications

Most frequent side effects | Patient teaching

ANTIRETROVIRALS

Terminates viral replication.
NRTI:
Nucleoside reverse transcriptase inhibitor
zidovudine (Retrovir)
Blocks enzyme activity.
NNRTI:
Nonnucleoside reverse transcriptase inhibitor
efavirenz (Sustiva)
Inhibits and prevents maturation of HIV.
PI:
Protease inhibitor
saquinavir (Invirase)
Highly active antiviral therapy (HAART) is treatment with three to four drugs.
Blocks viral entry and replication.
HIV-fusion inhibitor
enfuvirtide (Fuzeon)
Blocks viral entry.
CCR5 antagonist
maraviroc (Selzentry)
JMILLER

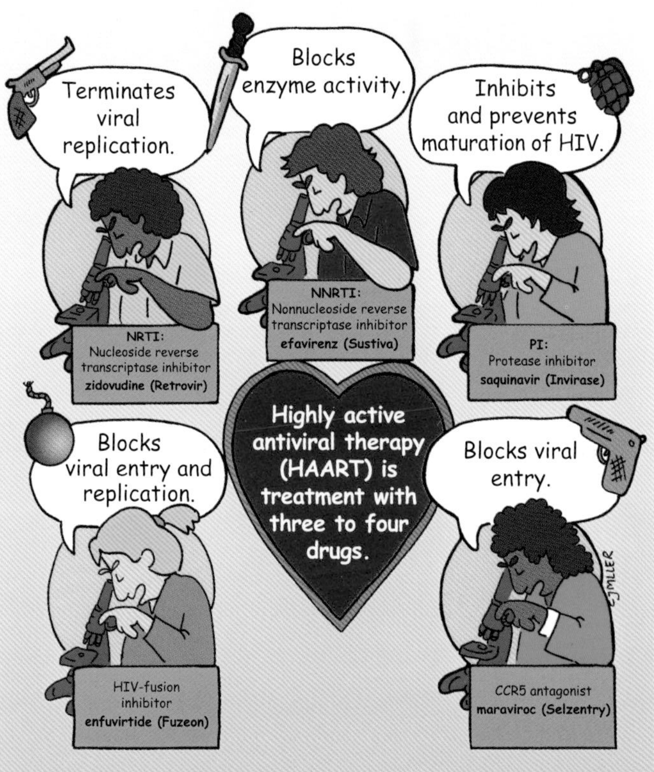

What You Need to Know

ANTIRETROVIRALS

Actions

- Nucleoside/nucleotide reverse transcriptase inhibitors (NRTIs)—inhibits enzymes required for human immunodeficiency virus (HIV) replication
- Nonnucleoside reverse transcriptase inhibitors (NNRTIs)—disrupt enzyme activity
- Protease inhibitor (PI)—inhibits enzyme activity and prevents maturation of virus
- HIV fusion inhibitor—blocks entry of virus into CD4-T cells
- Chemokine receptor 5 antagonist (CCR5)—blocks viral entry; some strains of HIV require CCR5

Contraindications and Precautions

- Known hypersensitivity and/or intolerable toxicity

Side Effects

- *NRTI:* anemia and neutropenia from bone marrow suppression, GI upset; rarely lactic acidosis and hepatic steatosis (fatty liver)
- *NNRTI:* central nervous system (CNS) symptoms (dizziness, insomnia, drowsiness); rash may range from mild to severe; check liver function studies
- *PI:* hyperglycemia, fat maldistribution (pseudo-Cushing syndrome), hyperlipidemia, bone loss, elevation in serum transaminases (liver injury)
- *HIV-fusion inhibitor:* injection site reactions, pneumonia, hypersensitivity
- *CCR5 antagonist:* cough, dizziness, pyrexia, rash, abdominal pain

Nursing Implications

1. Check to see whether medication should be taken with or without food because this varies with drug classes.
2. Instruct patient to take the full dose and complete treatment regimen.
3. Pregnant women should receive antiretroviral therapy regardless of pregnancy status.
4. Teach patient to report symptoms related to severe rash, CNS issues, elevated blood sugar, pneumonia.
5. Monitor CD4-T cell count—medications do not cure or kill HIV but slow replication.

Remember, **vir** at the start, middle, or end of a word means virus: acyclo**vir**, efa**vir**enz, enfu**vir**tide, Retro**vir**, saquina**vir** (In**vir**ase), mara**vir**oc.

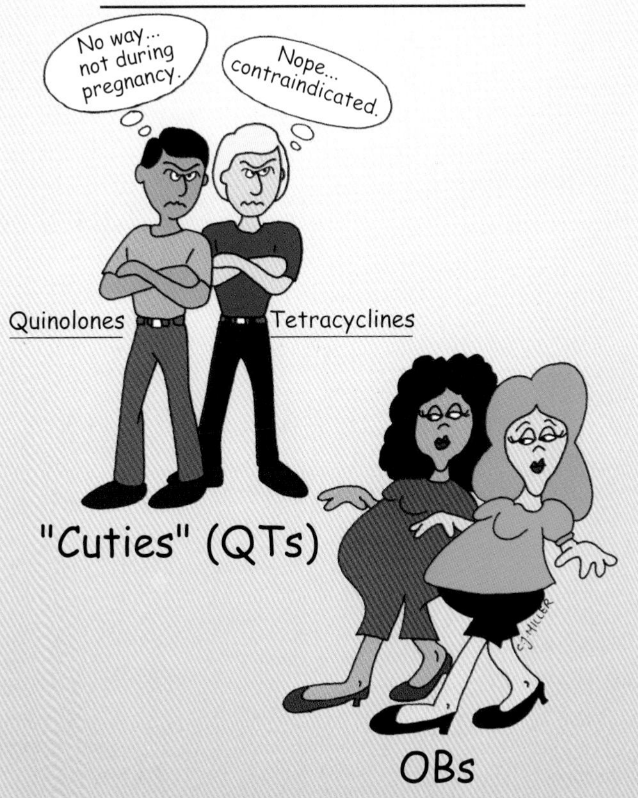
TWO QTs SAY NO TO OBs
No way... not during pregnancy.
Nope... contraindicated.
Quinolones
Tetracyclines
"Cuties" (QTs)
OBs
CJ MILLER

What You Need to Know

QUINOLONES AND TETRACYCLINES—DRUG IMPACT ON PREGNANCIES

FDA Pregnancy Risk Categories

- Category A: Remote risk of fetal harm
- Category B: Slightly more risk than category A
- Category C: Greater risk than category B
- Category D: Proven risk of fetal harm; labeled as warning
- Category X: Proven risk of fetal harm; labeled as contraindicated

Contraindications

- Women who are pregnant need to take a cautious approach to drug therapy during pregnancy. The health care provider is responsible for ordering medications that are safe and appropriate for the ever-changing physiologic dynamics during pregnancy.
- Contraindicated medications can cause detrimental changes in the mother, fetus, and fetal environment.
- Quinolones (category C) and tetracyclines (category D) are not routinely used during pregnancy.

Nursing Implications

1. Evaluate patient's level of understanding about her physiologic, mental, and emotional conditions.
2. Teach patient to call the prenatal clinic or physician's office before using any over-the-counter medications.
3. The patient should not take any medications that have not been specifically approved or prescribed by her health care provider.
4. Advise patient to avoid all alcoholic beverages during the term of the pregnancy.
5. Advise patient to report any unusual signs or symptoms of reactions to the treatment plan.

Think of the mnemonic **MCAT** to remember other antibiotics contraindicated in pregnancy. **M**—**M**etronidazole (contraindicated in first trimester; category B—second and third trimesters); **C**—**C**hloramphenicol (category C); **A**—**A**minoglycoside (category C): **T**—**T**etracycline (category D)

Important nursing implications | Serious/life-threatening implications

Most frequent side effects | Patient teaching

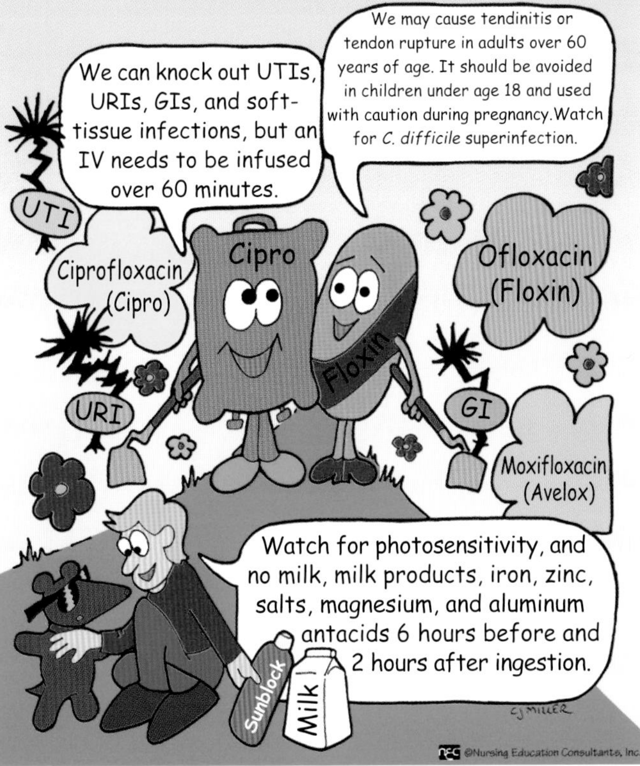
FLUOROQUINOLONES
We can knock out UTIs, URIs, GIs, and soft-tissue infections, but an IV needs to be infused over 60 minutes.
We may cause tendinitis or tendon rupture in adults over 60 years of age. It should be avoided in children under age 18 and used with caution during pregnancy. Watch for C. difficile superinfection.
UTI
Ciprofloxacin (Cipro)
Cipro
Floxin
Ofloxacin (Floxin)
URI
GI
Moxifloxacin (Avelox)
Watch for photosensitivity, and no milk, milk products, iron, zinc, salts, magnesium, and aluminum antacids 6 hours before and 2 hours after ingestion.
Sunblock
Milk
CJ MILLER
©Nursing Education Consultants, Inc.

What You Need to Know

FLUOROQUINOLONES

Classification

Antibacterial

Actions

Bactericidal; inhibits DNA enzyme that interferes with replication; is considered broad spectrum against most gram-negative and some gram-positive bacteria, but not against anaerobic infections.

Uses

- Respiratory, urinary, GI, bone, joint, skin, and soft-tissue infections
- Preferred drug for treatment of inhaled anthrax

Contraindications and Precautions

- Hypersensitivity, history of myasthenia gravis
- Children younger than age 18 years (systemic treatment should be avoided)
- Pregnancy

Side Effects

- GI upset—nausea, vomiting, diarrhea, abdominal pain
- Dizziness, headache, restlessness
- Patients older than 60 years, patients taking glucocorticoids, and patients who have undergone a heart, liver, or kidney transplantation are at highest risk for tendinitis and tendon rupture.
- Photosensitivity reactions: patients should avoid sunlight and sunlamps.
- Avoid moxifloxacin in patients with prolonged QT interval and hypokalemia.

Nursing Implications

1. Teach patient to avoid antacids, iron supplements, and milk and dairy products for at least 6 hours after taking medication; encourage adequate fluid intake.
2. Teach patient to report any tendon pain or inflammation.
3. Ciprofloxacin, norfloxacin, and ofloxacin can increase warfarin levels—monitor prothrombin (PT) time in patients taking warfarin.
4. Administer intravenous (IV) fluroquinolone medications over 60 minutes.
5. All oral medication dosing can be done with or without food, except for norfloxacin, which needs administered on an empty stomach.
6. Monitor for prolonged QT interval in cardiac patients taking antidysrhythmic medications.
7. Teach patient to wear sunscreen and protective clothing when in sunlight.

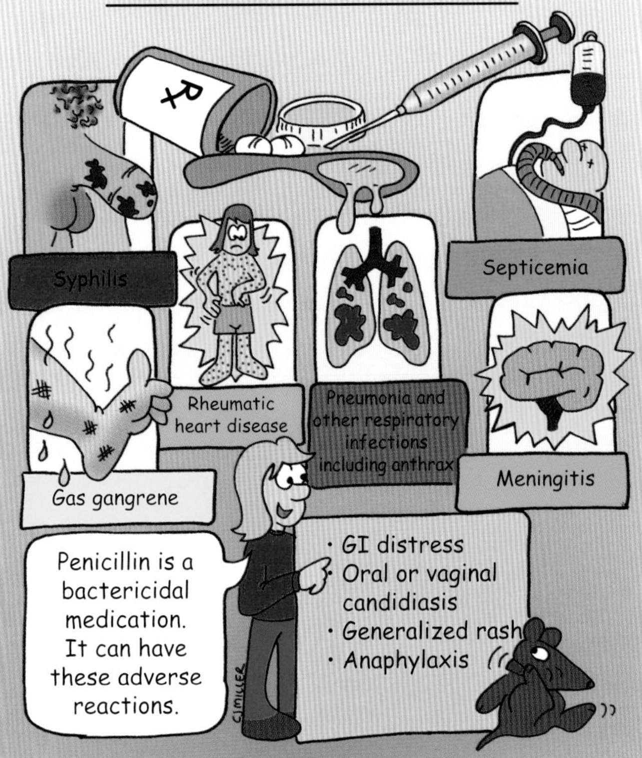
PENICILLIN (PCN)
USES AND SIDE EFFECTS
Syphilis
Septicemia
Rheumatic heart disease
Pneumonia and other respiratory infections including anthrax
Meningitis
Gas gangrene
Penicillin is a bactericidal medication. It can have these adverse reactions.
· GI distress
· Oral or vaginal candidiasis
· Generalized rash
· Anaphylaxis
CJMILLER

What You Need to Know

PENICILLIN (PCN)

Action

Bactericidal; disrupts and weakens the cell wall, leading to cell lysis and death

Use

Based on type of penicillin, treatment of infections caused by bacteria

Types

- Narrow spectrum that are penicillinase *sensitive*—penicillin G (Bicillin), penicillin V
- Narrow spectrum penicillinase *resistant* (antistaphylococcal penicillins)—nafcillin, oxacillin, dicloxacillin
- Broad-spectrum (aminopenicillins)—ampicillin, amoxicillin, amoxicillin/clavulanate (Augmentin)
- Extended-spectrum penicillins (antipseudomonal penicillins)—ticarcillin/clavulanate (Timentin), piperacillin/tazobactam (Zosyn)

Contraindications and Precautions

- Hypersensitivity or any history of allergic reaction to penicillin
- Caution in patients with allergy to cephalosporin, depending on severity of allergic response

Side Effects

- Allergic response (all types)—rash, itching, hives, anaphylaxis
- With ticarcillin—sodium overload (heart failure), and bleeding as a result of the interference with platelet function

Nursing Implications

1. Instruct patient to check label with regard to administering with food.
2. Instruct patient to wear medication-alert bracelet if allergic to penicillin.
3. Monitor renal and cardiac function and electrolyte levels to avoid toxic levels.
4. Monitor patient for 30 minutes when given parenterally; administer epinephrine if anaphylaxis occurs.
5. Collect any laboratory culture specimens before initiating penicillin therapy.
6. Do not mix aminoglycosides with penicillin in the same IV infusion—deactivates the aminoglycoside.
7. Monitor for circulatory overload and bleeding tendencies when patient receives ticarcillin/clavulanate.

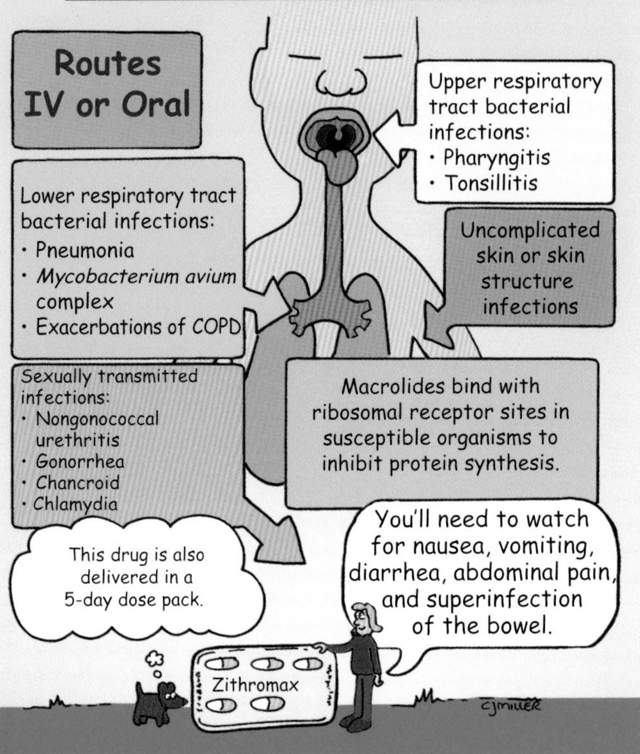
MACROLIDES
Top to Bottom...Mild to Moderate
Routes IV or Oral
Upper respiratory tract bacterial infections:
• Pharyngitis
• Tonsillitis
Lower respiratory tract bacterial infections:
• Pneumonia
• *Mycobacterium avium* complex
• Exacerbations of COPD
Uncomplicated skin or skin structure infections
Sexually transmitted infections:
• Nongonococcal urethritis
• Gonorrhea
• Chancroid
• Chlamydia
Macrolides bind with ribosomal receptor sites in susceptible organisms to inhibit protein synthesis.
This drug is also delivered in a 5-day dose pack.
You'll need to watch for nausea, vomiting, diarrhea, abdominal pain, and superinfection of the bowel.
Zithromax
CJMILLER

What You Need to Know

MACROLIDES

Action

Broad-spectrum antibiotic that binds with ribosomal receptor sites in susceptible organisms to inhibit bacterial protein synthesis.

Uses

- There are 3 main drugs:
  - Erythromycin
  - Azithromycin
  - Clarithromycin
- Treats upper respiratory tract, ear, and skin infections; syphilis (for penicillin-sensitive patients); cholera; and chancroid
- Azithromycin is drug of choice for *Chlamydia trachomatis*

Contraindications and Precautions

- Liver dysfunction.
- Avoid macrolides in patients with preexisting QT prolongation, and in those taking drugs that can increase erythromycin levels (e.g., verapamil, dilitiazem, HIV protease inhibitors, and azole antifungal drugs).

Side Effects

- Diarrhea, nausea and vomiting, abdominal pain.
- High levels of all forms of erythromycin can prolong the QT interval, thereby posing a risk of potentially fatal cardiac dysrhythmias.

Nursing Implications

1. Take medication 1 hour before or 2 hours after food or antacids.
2. Aluminum and magnesium antacids reduce rate of absorption but not extent.
3. Observe for development of signs of superinfection.
4. Instruct patient to take prescribed course of therapy, although symptoms may improve or disappear.
5. IV preparations are infused slowly over 60 minutes.
6. Patients taking erythromycin and all of its forms—monitor warfarin levels and watch for prolonged QT interval.

Important nursing implications | Serious/life-threatening implications

Most frequent side effects | Patient teaching

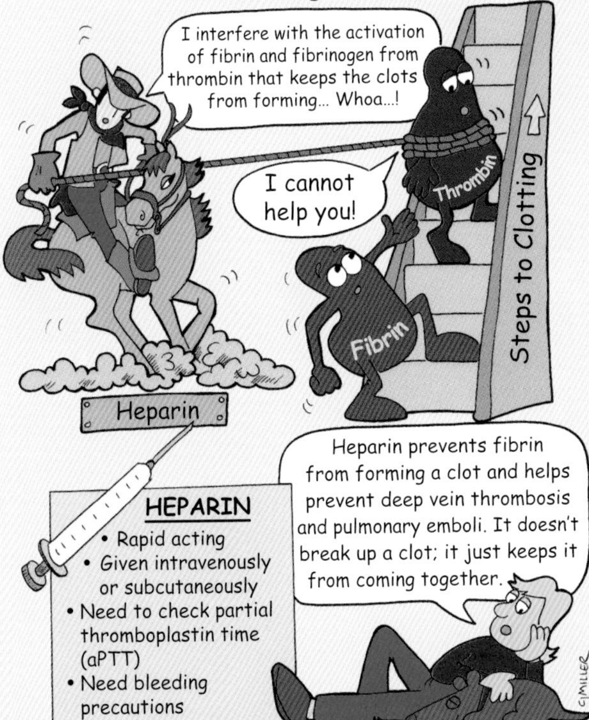
HEPARIN
The Clotting Roundup
I interfere with the activation of fibrin and fibrinogen from thrombin that keeps the clots from forming... Whoa...!
I cannot help you!
Thrombin
Steps to Clotting
Fibrin
Heparin
HEPARIN
• Rapid acting
• Given intravenously or subcutaneously
• Need to check partial thromboplastin time (aPTT)
• Need bleeding precautions
Heparin prevents fibrin from forming a clot and helps prevent deep vein thrombosis and pulmonary emboli. It doesn't break up a clot; it just keeps it from coming together.
GJMILLER

What You Need to Know

HEPARIN

Action

Heparin is an anticoagulant that exerts a direct effect on blood coagulation by enhancing the inhibitory actions of antithrombin on several factors essential to normal blood clotting, thereby blocking the conversion of prothrombin to thrombin and fibrinogen to fibrin.

Uses

- Rapid acting (within minutes) to prevent and treat deep vein thrombosis (DVT), pulmonary embolism, and emboli in atrial fibrillation
- Used to treat disseminated intravascular coagulation (DIC)
- Is preferred anticoagulant during pregnancy (doesn't cross the placenta or enter breast milk)
- Prevents coagulation in heart-lung machines and dialyzers in patients after open-heart surgery and dialysis
- Used as an adjunct to thrombolytic therapy of acute myocardial infarction (MI)

Precautions and Contraindications

- Bleeding tendencies—hemophilia, dissecting aneurysm, peptic ulcer
- Thrombocytopenia, uncontrollable bleeding, threatened abortion
- Postoperative patients—especially eye, brain, and spinal cord surgeries; lumbar puncture; and regional anesthesia

Side Effects

- Injection site reactions and heparin-induced thrombocytopenia may develop.
- May result in spontaneous bleeding.

Nursing Implications

1. Monitor partial thromboplastin time (PTT) and activated PTT (aPTT)—should be 1½ to 2 times the control value. *Watch for bleeding.*
2. May not be given orally, or by intramuscular (IM) injection; protamine sulfate is the antidote.
3. Caution patients not to take aspirin or any medication that decreases platelet aggregation (clopidogrel) unless ordered specifically by health care provider.
4. Administered either intravenously (IV) or subcutaneously; apply firm pressure for 1 to 2 minutes; do not massage site after injection.
5. Dosage is prescribed in units, not milligrams (mg).

Important nursing implications	Serious/life-threatening implications
Most frequent side effects	Patient teaching

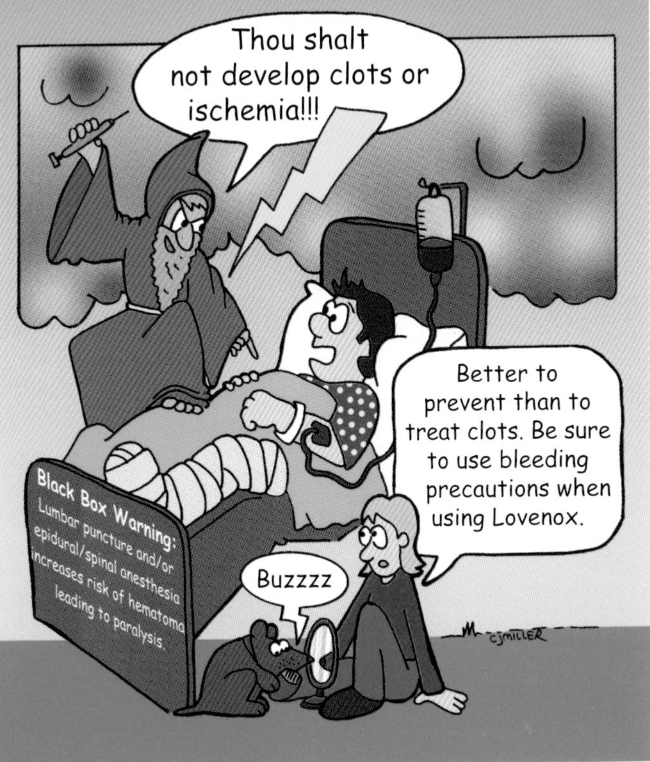
ENOXAPARIN (LOVENOX)
Thou shalt not develop clots or ischemia!!!
Better to prevent than to treat clots. Be sure to use bleeding precautions when using Lovenox.
Black Box Warning:
Lumbar puncture and/or epidural/spinal anesthesia increases risk of hematoma leading to paralysis.
Buzzzz
CJMILLER

What You Need to Know

ENOXAPARIN (LOVENOX)

Actions

Low–molecular-weight heparin (LMWH) with a great affinity for factor Xa in providing anticoagulation action; provides a predictable anticoagulant response

Uses

Prevention of postoperative deep vein thrombosis, pulmonary embolism; prevention of ischemic complications in unstable angina, or non–Q-wave myocardial infarction (MI), and ST-elevation MI (STEMI)

Contraindications

- Presence of any active bleeding
- Increased risk of hematoma in patients with spinal or epidural anesthesia
- Use with caution with concurrent use of aspirin, clopidogrel, and other antiplatelet medications
- Not to be used in presence of thrombocytopenia

Side Effects

- Immune-mediated thrombocytopenia
- Bleeding episodes

Nursing Implications

1. Medication is only administered subcutaneously.
2. Protamine sulfate is antidote.
3. Always double-check—cannot be given to a patient receiving heparin.
4. Injections in abdomen should be 2 inches from umbilicus or any incisional area.
5. Advise patient not to take any over-the-counter (OTC) medications, especially aspirin.
6. Check complete blood count (CBC), especially platelet count.
7. Monitor for bleeding:
   - Guaiac stools for occult blood
   - Hematuria
   - Bleeding gums
   - Excessive bruising
8. Does not require activated partial thromboplastin time (aPTT) monitoring.

Important nursing implications | Serious/life-threatening implications
Most frequent side effects | Patient teaching

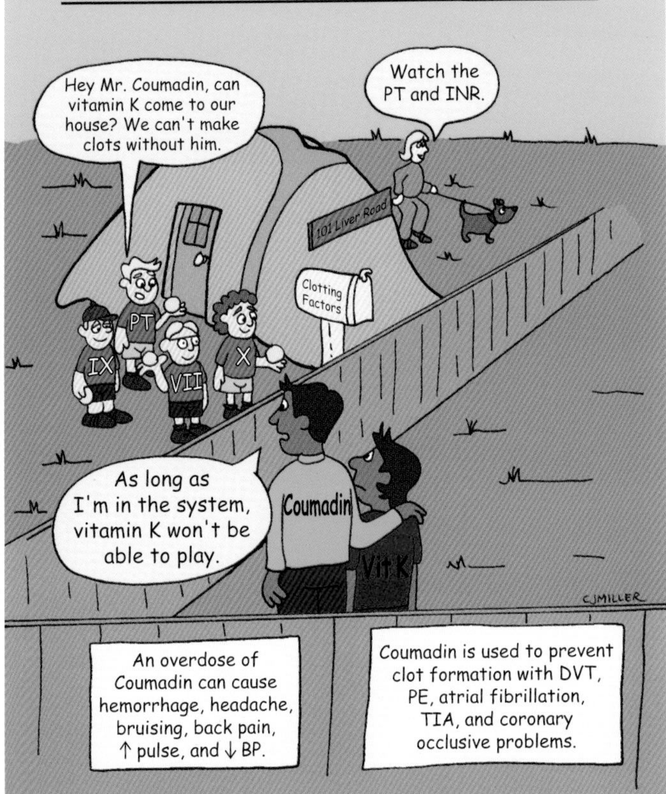
WARFARIN SODIUM (COUMADIN)
Hey Mr. Coumadin, can vitamin K come to our house? We can't make clots without him.
Watch the PT and INR.
101 Liver Road
Clotting Factors
PT
IX
VII
X
As long as I'm in the system, vitamin K won't be able to play.
Coumadin
Vit K
CJMILLER
An overdose of Coumadin can cause hemorrhage, headache, bruising, back pain, ↑ pulse, and ↓ BP.
Coumadin is used to prevent clot formation with DVT, PE, atrial fibrillation, TIA, and coronary occlusive problems.

What You Need to Know

WARFARIN SODIUM (COUMADIN)

Actions

Warfarin is an oral anticoagulant that antagonizes vitamin K, which is necessary for the synthesis of clotting factors VII, IX, X, and prothrombin. As a result, it disrupts the coagulation cascade.

Uses

- Long-term prophylaxis of thrombosis; is not useful in emergency because of delayed onset of action
- Prevents venous thrombosis and thromboembolism associated with atrial fibrillation and prosthetic heart valves
- Decreases risk of recurrent transient ischemic attacks (TIAs) and recurrent myocardial infarction

Contraindications

- Bleeding disorders (hemophilia, thrombocytopenia)
- Lumbar puncture; regional anesthesia; or surgery of the eye, brain, or spinal cord
- Vitamin K deficiency; severe hypertension
- Pregnancy—category X; breast-feeding (crosses into breast milk)
- Liver disease, alcoholism

Side Effects

- Spontaneous bleeding
- Hypersensitivity reactions (e.g., dermatitis, fever, pruritus, urticaria)
- Red-orange discoloration of urine (not to be confused with hematuria); weakening of bones with long-term use leading to risk of fractures

Nursing Implications

1. Monitor prothrombin time (PT) and international normalized ratio (INR) as ordered (2 to 3 is usually an acceptable INR for anticoagulation).
2. Interacts with a large number of medications; consequently, evaluate medications for interactions before initiating therapy.
3. Monitor for bleeding tendencies; vitamin K is an antidote.
4. Teach patient to maintain intake of vitamin K (keep constant intake of foods such as green, leafy vegetables, mayonnaise, and canola oil) and do not abruptly increase or decrease intake.
5. Patient must advise all health care providers if patient is taking warfarin, because it is very slow to be excreted from the body.
6. Teach patient to wear a medical alert bracelet.

EPOETIN ALFA (PROCRIT)

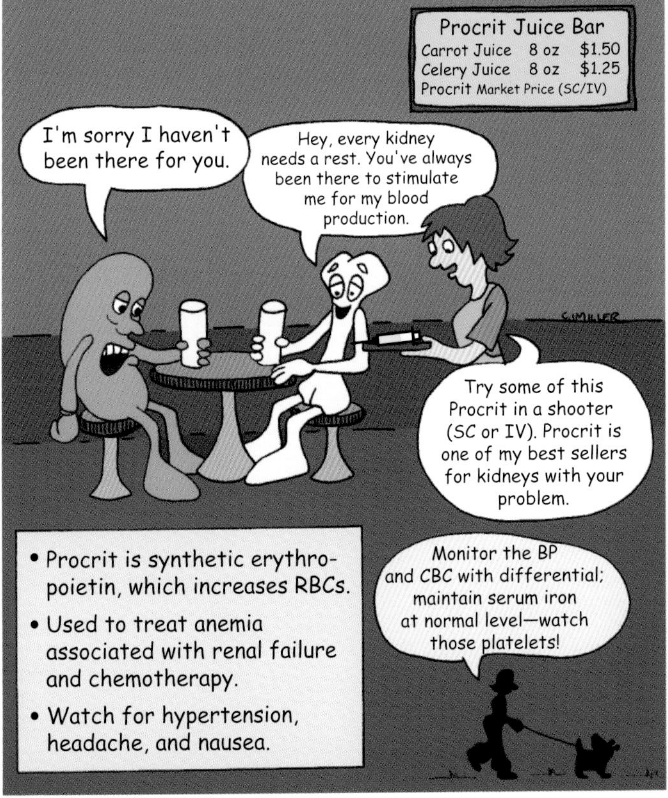

Procrit Juice Bar
Carrot Juice 8 oz $1.50
Celery Juice 8 oz $1.25
Procrit Market Price (SC/IV)

I'm sorry I haven't been there for you.

Hey, every kidney needs a rest. You've always been there to stimulate me for my blood production.

Try some of this Procrit in a shooter (SC or IV). Procrit is one of my best sellers for kidneys with your problem.

- Procrit is synthetic erythropoietin, which increases RBCs.
- Used to treat anemia associated with renal failure and chemotherapy.
- Watch for hypertension, headache, and nausea.

Monitor the BP and CBC with differential; maintain serum iron at normal level—watch those platelets!

What You Need to Know

EPOETIN ALFA (PROCRIT)

Action

Erythropoietic growth factor that stimulates red blood cell production in the bone marrow

Uses

- Patients with anemia as a result of chronic renal failure, chemotherapy
- Patients infected with human immunodeficiency virus (HIV) and taking zidovudine (Retrovir)
- Patients with anemia before elective surgery

Contraindications

- Hemoglobin in excess of 11 mg/dL; hypersensitivity to albumin

Precautions

- Poorly controlled hypertension; hypersensitivity to albumin
- Patients with cancers of myeloid origin

Side Effects

- Hypertension
- Cardiovascular events—cardiac arrest, heart failure, thrombotic events (stroke, myocardial infarction [MI])
- Patients with cancer—tumor progression and shortened survival
- Autoimmune pure red-cell aplasia (PRCA)—severe anemia, red blood cell (RBC) production ceases (rarely occurs)

Nursing Implications

1. Monitor blood pressure before erythropoietin therapy.
2. Do not shake solution; it may denature the glycoprotein. Do not mix with other medications.
3. Discard remaining contents because erythropoietin does not contain a preservative.
4. Monitor hematocrit (Hct), hemoglobin (Hb), and serum iron levels as well as fluid and electrolyte balance.
5. Monitor for seizures (rapid increase in Hct level increases risk of hypertensive encephalopathy).
6. Provide patient with required *Medication Guide* from the Food and Drug Administration (FDA).

Important nursing implications | Serious/life-threatening implications

Most frequent side effects | Patient teaching

IRON SUPPLEMENTS

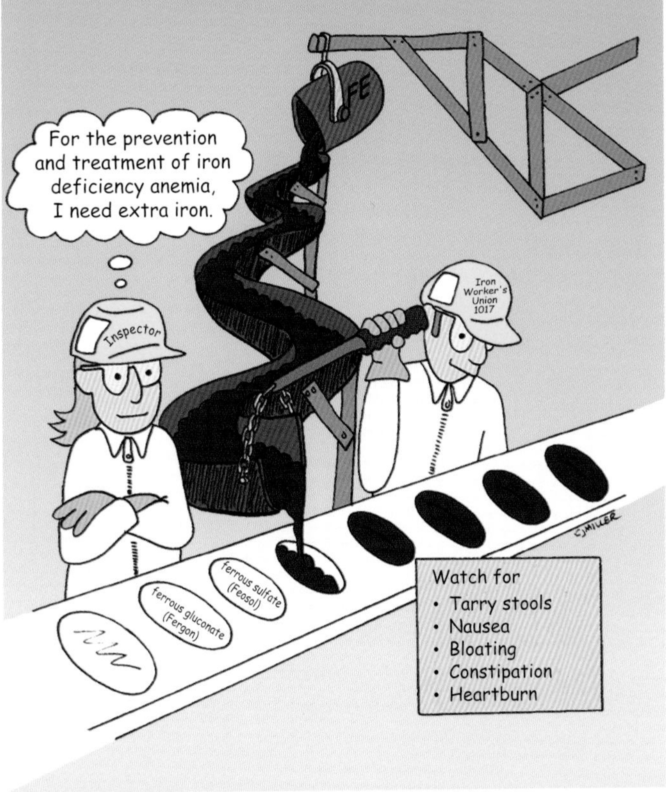

FE

For the prevention and treatment of iron deficiency anemia, I need extra iron.

Inspector

Iron Worker's Union 1017

ferrous sulfate (Feosol)

ferrous gluconate (Fergon)

Watch for
- Tarry stools
- Nausea
- Bloating
- Constipation
- Heartburn

What You Need to Know

IRON SUPPLEMENTS (ORAL FERROUS IRON SALTS)

Action

Hematinic agent used in the production of normal hemoglobin and red blood cells for transportation and utilization of oxygen

Uses

- Iron deficiency anemia (microcytic, hypochromic)
- Prophylactic use in pregnancy and childhood

Contraindications and Precautions

- All anemias other than iron deficiency anemia
- Peptic ulcers, regional enteritis, colitis
- Iron-containing products are leading cause of iron poisoning in young children.

Side Effects

- Gastrointestinal (GI) disturbances—nausea (usually transient), heartburn (pyrosis), bloating, constipation
- Tarry stools or dark-green discoloration (not associated with bleeding)
- Iron toxicity due to accidental or intentional overdose (usually in children and not with therapeutic doses)

Nursing Implications

1. Do not give with antacids or tetracyclines, or crush or chew sustained-release medications.
2. Take between meals to maximize uptake.
3. Take vitamin C (ascorbic acid) to promote the absorption of the iron.
4. Because liquid preparations stain teeth, use a straw or dilute; follow with rinsing the mouth.
5. Teach patient that oral iron supplements differ from one another and should not be interchanged.
6. Diet teaching to include iron-rich foods—liver, eggs, meat, fish, and fowl.
7. Teach to store iron out of reach and in childproof containers; iron poisoning can be fatal to young children.
8. Parenteral deferoxamine (Desferal) and the oral drug deferasirox (Exjade) are used for chronic iron overload caused by blood transfusions—drugs absorb iron and prevent toxic effects.

Important nursing implications	Serious/life-threatening implications
Most frequent side effects	Patient teaching

THROMBOLYTICS

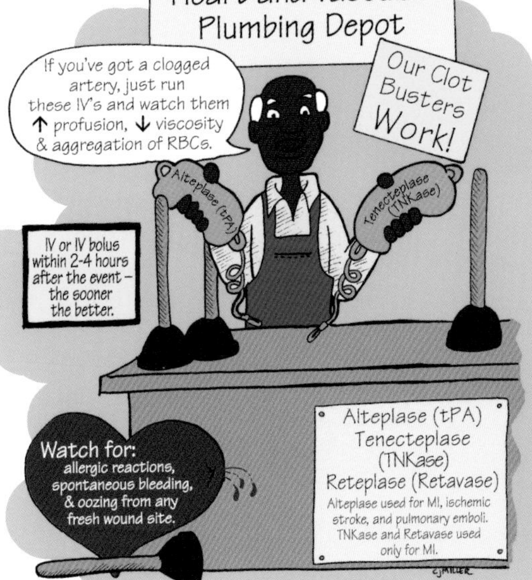

What You Need to Know

THROMBOLYTICS

Actions

Work to directly or indirectly convert plasminogen to plasmin, an enzyme that acts to digest the fibrin matrix of clots. Dissolve existing thrombi rather than prevent them from occurring. Also known as *fibrinolytics* or informally as *clot busters*—alteplase (tPA), tenecteplase (TNKase), reteplace (Retavase).

Uses

- All three medications used in treatment of acute myocardial infarction
- tPA used also for pulmonary embolism, acute ischemic stroke, and restoring patency in a clogged central venous catheter

Contraindications and Precautions

- Cerebrovascular disease and pregnancy
- Active internal bleeding, aortic dissection, history of poorly controlled hypertension
- Any prior intracranial hemorrhage or recent head injury
- Recent major surgery or trauma within the prior 2 to 4 weeks
- History of gastrointestinal (GI) bleeding
- Ischemic stroke within the prior 6 months

Side Effects

- Hemorrhage (intracranial of greatest concern) and anemia
- Bleeding from recent wounds and needle punctures
- Hypersensitivity reactions—itching, urticaria, headache
- Hypotension, cardiac dysrhythmias

Nursing Implications

1. Administer immediately after the event for better outcome, preferably within 2 to 4 hours.
2. Monitor intake and output and hematocrit levels during treatment.
3. Monitor patient for bleeding and hypersensitivity reactions.
4. While receiving the medication, maintain patient on bed rest; avoid subcutaneous (SQ) and intramuscular (IM) injections.

Important nursing implications | Serious/life-threatening implications

Most frequent side effects | Patient teaching

CLOPIDOGREL (PLAVIX)

"When platelets gather together, use Plavix for crowd control."

Platelets for peaceful aggregation!
We have rights!
We can't stick together now that we're apart!
PLAVIX
PLAVIX
All right...break it up! No gathering when we (Plavix) are around.

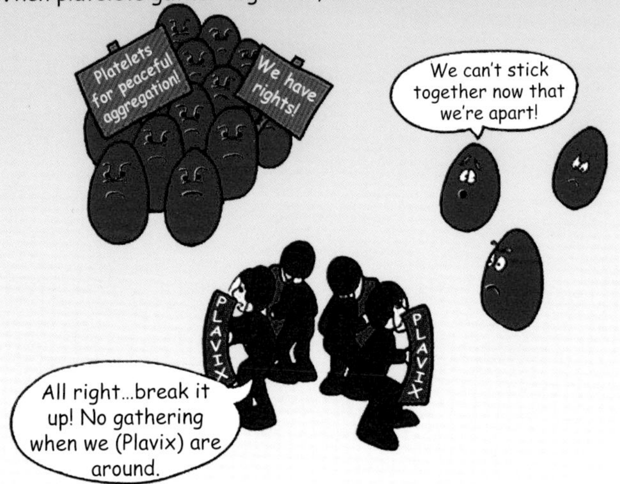

Plavix works by inhibiting platelet aggregation. It is used to decrease the incidence of vascular clotting, MIs, stroke, and acute coronary syndrome.

Watch for rash and GI upset. Use with caution with hepatic and renal problems and with a history of bleeding.

Check platelet counts before beginning, then weekly.

What You Need to Know

CLOPIDOGREL (PLAVIX)

Classification

Antiplatelet

Action

Suppresses platelet aggregation in arterial circulation; antiplatelet action occurs within 2 hours of administration.

Uses

- Prevent occlusion of coronary stents
- Prevent/reduce thrombotic problems, such as myocardial infarction (MI), ischemic stroke, peripheral arterial disorders
- Secondary prevention of atherothrombotic events in patients with acute coronary syndromes (ACS), defined as unstable angina or MI

Contraindications and Precautions

- Active bleeding
- Hypersensitivity, breast-feeding, renal and hepatic disease

Side Effects

- Abdominal pain, dyspepsia, diarrhea (concern with gastrointestinal [GI] bleeding)
- Bleeding—epistaxis, purpura
- Rash

Nursing Implications

1. May administer with food to diminish GI upset.
2. Teach patient to report any unusual bleeding or bruising (hematuria, tarry stools, epistaxis).
3. Teach patient that if surgery is scheduled, medication may be held 5 days before surgery.
4. Platelet counts may be monitored.
5. Patient should notify all health care providers regarding the medication.
6. Should not be taken with proton pump inhibitors—omeprazole (Prilosec); unless the patient has risk factors for GI bleeding (advanced age, use of non-steroidal antiinflammatory drugs [NSAIDs] or anticoagulants), the benefits of combining a proton pump inhibitor (PPI) with clopidogrel usually outweigh any risk from reduced antiplatelet effects.

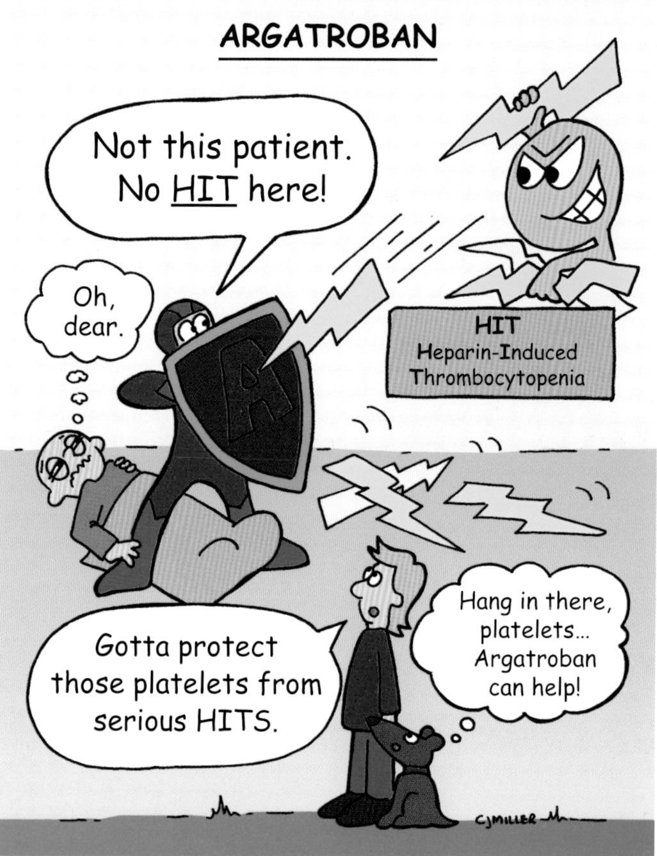
ARGATROBAN
Not this patient. No HIT here!
Oh, dear.
HIT
Heparin-Induced
Thrombocytopenia
Gotta protect those platelets from serious HITS.
Hang in there, platelets... Argatroban can help!
CJMILLER

What You Need to Know

ARGATROBAN

Classification

Anticoagulant

Action

Directly inhibits the action of thrombin in the clotting mechanism

Uses

Prevents and treats heparin-induced thrombocytopenia (HIT); prevents HIT during coronary procedures

Contraindication

- Any evidence of overt bleeding

Precautions

- Severe hypertension, hepatic impairment (dose adjusted)
- Recent major surgery
- Spinal anesthesia or lumbar puncture
- History of any bleeding disorders or intracranial bleeding

Side Effects

- Allergic reactions: dyspnea, cough, rash—primarily in patients receiving other thrombolytic drugs or contrast media
- Hypotension, fever, diarrhea
- Bleeding episodes—hematuria, epistaxis, tarry stools, petechiae

Nursing Implications

1. Carefully monitor patient for any evidence of bleeding.
2. Monitor platelet count.
3. Administer only intravenously (IV)
4. Dose and rate of administration are based on body weight.
5. Obtain baseline activated partial prothrombin time (aPTT) to monitor treatment. The aPTT returns to base level in 2 to 4 hours after medication is stopped. Dosage is adjusted to maintain the aPTT at 1.5 to 3 times the baseline value.

Important nursing implications | Serious/life-threatening implications

Most frequent side effects | Patient teaching

ANTICOAGULANTS FOR ATRIAL FIBRILLATION

Rivaroxaban (Xarelto) and Dabigatran (Pradaxa)

I am in atrial fibrillation.

No way clots! We will keep you from forming!

Quick, let's form clots!

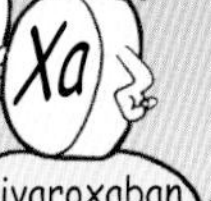

XIII

Rivaroxaban (Xarelto)

Dabigatran (Pradaxa)

- Prevents strokes
- Rapid onset
- Fewer bleeding problems
- Fixed oral dosage
- Fewer drug interactions

Taken by mouth, they may cause dyspepsia, but no blood test (INR) monitoring is required.

Dyspepsia... Sounds like a diet cola.

CJ MILLER

What You Need to Know

Anticoagulants for Atrial Fibrillation

DABIGATRAN; RIVAROXABAN; APIXABAN; EDOXABAN

Classification

Anticoagulant

Dabigatran (Pradaxa): direct thrombin inhibitor
Rivaroxaban (Xarelto): direct factor Xa inhibitor
Apixaban (Eliquis): direct factor Xa inhibitor
Edoxaban (Savaysa): direct factor Xa inhibitor

Action

Dabigatran

Directly inhibits thrombin formation, prevents conversion of fibrinogen to fibrin, prevents activation of factor XIII, and prevents the conversion of soluble fibrin into insoluble fibrin.

Rivaroxaban, apixaban, edoxaban

Inhibits production of thrombin by binding directly with factor Xa

Uses

Prevent strokes and systemic embolism in patients with atrial fibrillation that is not related to a cardiac valve problem

Precautions

- Pregnancy, active bleeding episodes
- Patients undergoing spinal puncture and/or epidural anesthesia
- Should not be combined with other anticoagulants; concurrent use with antiplatelet drugs and fibrinolytics should be done with caution (especially with rivaroxaban)
- Patients with severe renal or hepatic disease

Side Effects

- Bleeding, gastrointestinal [GI] disturbances—dyspepsia, gastritis-like syndrome (with dabigatran)

Nursing Implications

1. Does not require monitoring by activated partial prothrombin time (aPTT) or international normalized ratio (INR) levels.
2. Evaluate and monitor patient for bleeding risks.
3. Patient should take a missed dose as soon as possible, but not within 6 hours of next scheduled dose.
4. Dabigatran—after container is opened, medication should be used within 30 days; it is sensitive to moisture and should not be stored in weekly pill organizers.
5. Take with food to decrease gastric side effects

ANTIHYPERTENSIVES

Welcome, sports fans, to the super bowl of hypertension...
Coach
Play Book
Watch for hypotension, peripheral edema, flushing, headache, and GI upset. Now, get in there and play!
CA
CA
CA
CA
amlodipine (Norvasc)
verapamil (Calan)
nifedipine (Procardia)
diltiazem (Cardizem)
Blocking for the cardiac team will be the calcium channel blockers...
Watch for bradycardia hypotension, HF, broncho-spasms, and diminished sexual function.
Nobody quits these guys without seeing a doctor first!
BETA
BETA
BETA
BETA
metoprolol (Lopressor)
atenolol (Tenormin)
propranolol (Inderal)
nadolol (Corgard)
CJMILLER
The backup players for the cardiac team will be the beta-adrenergic blockers...

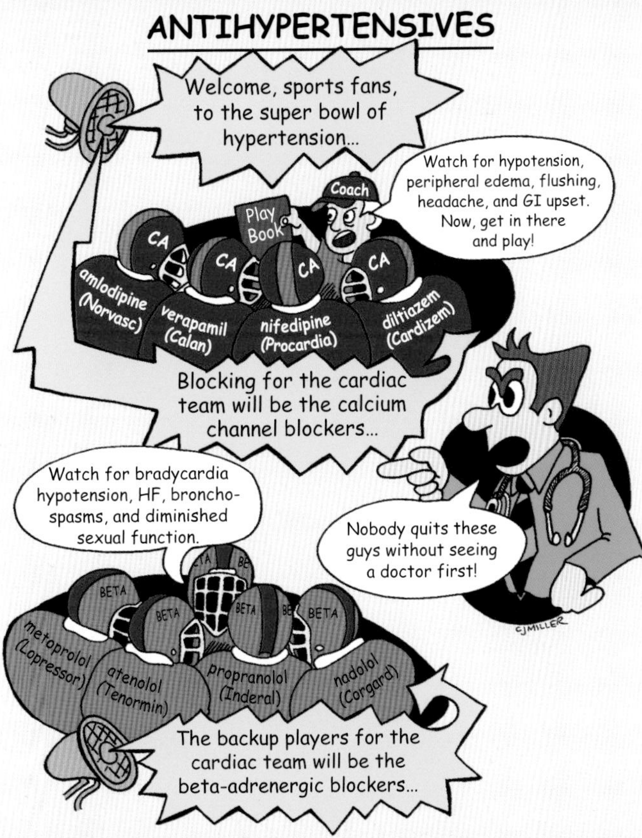

What You Need to Know

ANTIHYPERTENSIVES

Actions

Antihypertensive drugs act on the vascular, cardiac, renal, and sympathetic nervous systems. They also act to lower blood pressure (BP), cardiac output, and peripheral vascular resistance.

Uses

- Control hypertension
- Angina pectoris, cardiac dysrhythmias
- Hypertensive emergency

Contraindications

- Hypersensitivity
- Arterial stenosis
- Cerebrovascular insufficiency
- Severe bradycardia, AV heart block

Precautions

- Uncontrolled heart failure, thyrotoxicosis
- Beta-blockers can mask symptoms of hypoglycemia in patients with diabetes
- Hepatic and renal dysfunction

Side Effects

- Hypotension, sedation
- Calcium channel blockers—bradycardia, peripheral edema, constipation
- Beta-blockers—bradycardia, decreased atrioventricular (AV) conduction, reduced cardiac contractility, hypoglycemia, bronchoconstriction

Nursing Implications

1. Monitor vital signs.
2. Teach patients about orthostatic hypotension for initial dosing (e.g., get up slowly) and other lifestyle changes—weight reduction, sodium restriction, and daily exercise.
3. Monitor electrolyte, hepatic, and renal serum blood studies.
4. Avoid abrupt withdrawal of drug; may cause rebound phenomenon of excessive rise in BP.
5. Verapamil and diltiazem—do not drink grapefruit juice when taking medication.

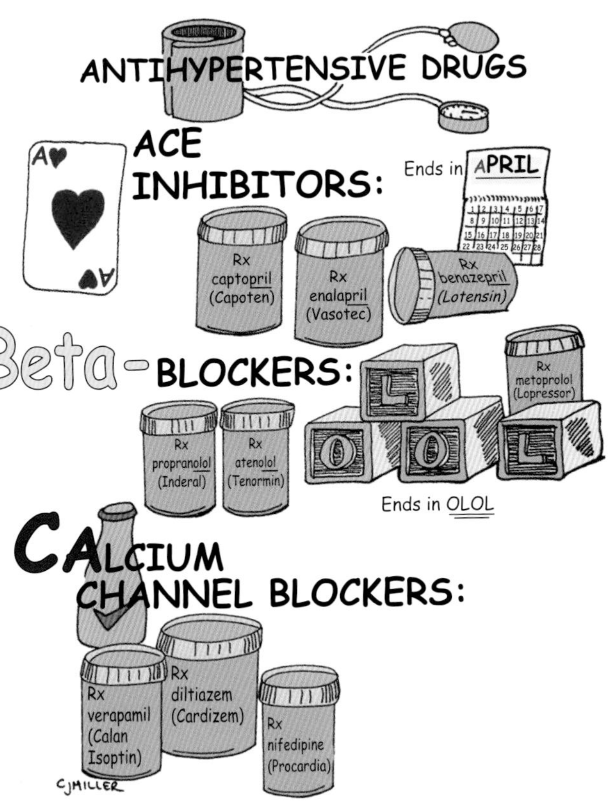
ANTIHYPERTENSIVE DRUGS
ACE
INHIBITORS:
Ends in APRIL
Rx
captopril
(Capoten)
Rx
enalapril
(Vasotec)
Rx
benazepril
(Lotensin)
Beta-BLOCKERS:
Rx
propranolol
(Inderal)
Rx
atenolol
(Tenormin)
Rx
metoprolol
(Lopressor)
Ends in OLOL
CALCIUM
CHANNEL BLOCKERS:
Rx
verapamil
(Calan
Isoptin)
Rx
diltiazem
(Cardizem)
Rx
nifedipine
(Procardia)
CJMILLER

What You Need to Know

ANTIHYPERTENSIVE DRUGS

Classification

Blood pressure is regulated by cardiac output (CO) and peripheral vascular resistance (PVR). Medications that influence either one of these systems lead to blood pressure control. Antihypertensive drugs that influence these systems to lower blood pressure are angiotensin-converting enzyme (ACE) inhibitors, beta-adrenergic blockers, and calcium channel blockers (CCBs).

Actions

- **A**—ACE inhibitors block the conversion of angiotensin I to angiotensin II, a vasoconstrictor. This block causes vasodilation and therefore decreases PVR, resulting in a decrease in blood pressure. Aldosterone is also blocked, causing a decrease in sodium and water retention.
- **B**—Beta-adrenergic blockers block the beta$_1$-receptors in the heart, which results in decreased heart rate and decreased force of contraction.
- **C**—CCBs block calcium influx into beta-receptors, decrease the force of myocardial contraction, reduce heart rate, and decrease PVR.

Uses

- Control hypertension
- Either as separate drugs or frequently in combination with another drug

Nursing Implications

1. Initial drug selection starts with a thiazide diuretic, typically followed by a beta-adrenergic blocker or an ACE inhibitor or CCB.
2. Take medication as prescribed; do not stop abruptly.
3. Teach patient never to double up on doses if a dose is missed.
4. Change positions slowly; watch for postural hypertension.
5. Avoid over-the-counter medications.
6. Take caution in hot weather, hot showers, hot tub baths, or prolonged sitting or standing because these may aggravate low blood pressure.
7. Teach patients about multidrug therapy; instruct them not to discontinue a previous antihypertensive medication when another medication is started.

Important nursing implications | Serious/life-threatening implications
Most frequent side effects | Patient teaching

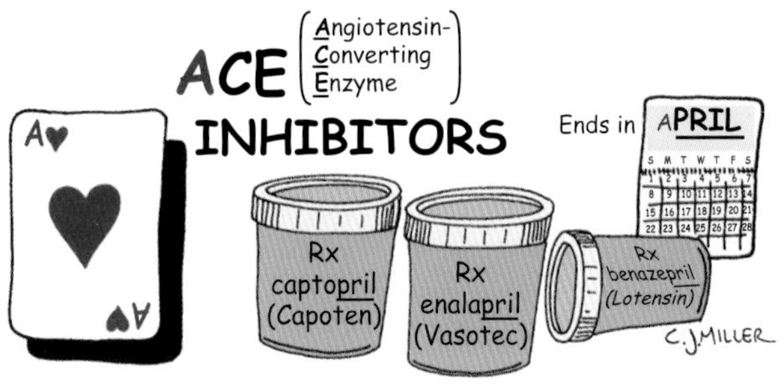

Actions: ↓ Peripheral vascular resistance **without:**

↑ Cardiac output
↑ Cardiac rate
↑ Cardiac contractility

Side Effects: Dizziness
Orthostatic hypotension
Fetal injury
Cough
Headache
Hyperkalemia

What You Need to Know

ANGIOTENSIN-CONVERTING ENZYME (ACE) INHIBITORS

Action

Blocks *production* of angiotensin II from the renin-angiotensin-aldosterone system, reduces peripheral resistance, and improves cardiac output

Uses

- Hypertension, heart failure, myocardial infarction (MI)
- Diabetic and nondiabetic nephropathy

CONTRAINDICATIONS

- History of angioedema
- Pregnancy
- Bilateral renal artery stenosis

Precautions

- Renal failure, collagen vascular disease
- Hypovolemia, salt depletion

Side Effects

- Postural hypotension (especially the first dose), headache, dizziness
- Nagging, dry, irritating, nonproductive cough
- Rash, angioedema
- Hyperkalemia
- Neutropenia (mainly with captopril)

Nursing Implications

1. Closely monitor blood pressure, especially for 2 hours after the first dose, because severe first-dose hypotension often develops.
2. Teach patient to rise slowly from a lying to a sitting position to reduce postural hypotensive effects.
3. Before administering, assess the patient for history or presence of renal impairment.
4. Administer on an empty stomach for best absorption.
5. Teach patient to notify health care provider if cough develops.
6. Teach patient to avoid potassium supplements or potassium-containing salt substitutes.
7. Monitor renal function and comblete blood count (CBC) and differential.

Important nursing implications — Serious/life-threatening implications

Most frequent side effects — Patient teaching

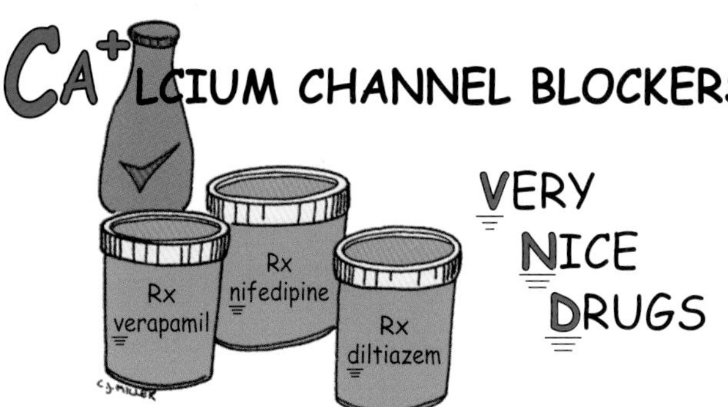

Actions: Blocks calcium access to cells causing:

- ↓ Contractility
- ↓ Conductivity of the heart
- ↓ Demand for oxygen

Side Effects:

- ↓ BP
- Bradycardia
- May precipitate AV block
- Headache
- Abdominal discomfort (constipation, nausea)
- Peripheral edema

What You Need to Know

CALCIUM CHANNEL BLOCKERS

Action

Block calcium access to the cells, causing decreased heart contractility and conductivity and leading to a decreased demand for oxygen; promote vasodilation.

Uses

- Angina, hypertension, and dysrhythmias (verapamil and diltiazem)

Contraindications

- *Nifedipine:* reflex tachycardia
- *Verapamil:* severe left ventricular dysfunction, decreased blood pressure, cardiogenic shock, or heart block
- *Diltiazem:* sick sinus syndrome, heart block, decreased blood pressure, acute myocardial infarction, or pulmonary congestion

Precautions

- Renal or hepatic insufficiency may develop.
- Avoid giving verapamil or diltiazem with beta-blockers and digoxin.

Side Effects

- Decreased blood pressure, edema of the extremities, headache
- Constipation (verapamil), nausea, skin flushing, dysrhythmias

Nursing Implications

1. Administer before meals; may be taken with food if needed; do not crush or allow patient to chew sustained-release medication preparations.
2. Monitor vital signs and watch for low blood pressure.
3. Teach about postural hypotension and to notify health care provider of signs of edema (swelling in ankles or feet).
4. Check liver and renal function studies.
5. Weigh patient; report any peripheral edema or weight gain.
6. Teach patient to avoid grapefruit juice.
7. Teach patient that constipation can be minimized by increasing dietary fiber and fluid.
8. Teach patients to notify health care provider of symptoms of slow heartbeat, shortness of breath, or weight gain.

Important nursing implications | Serious/life-threatening implications
Most frequent side effects | Patient teaching

ANGIOTENSIN II RECEPTOR BLOCKERS (ARBs)

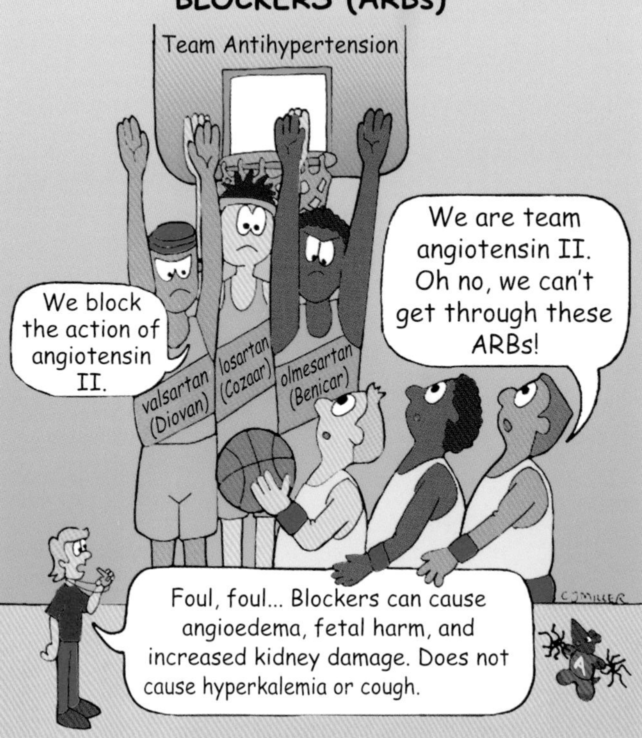

What You Need to Know

ANGIOTENSIN II RECEPTOR BLOCKERS (ARBs)

Actions

Blocks the *action*, but not the production, of angiotensin II. Blocks the access of angiotensin II to its receptors in heart, blood vessels, and adrenals, causing vasodilation.

Uses

- Hypertension
- Heart failure (valsartan, candesartan), myocardial infarction (MI) (valsartan)
- Diabetic neuropathy (irbesartan, losartan); retinopathy (losartan)
- Stroke prevention (losartan)
- Risk reduction in MI, stroke, death from cardiovascular causes in patients 55 years and older if intolerant to angiotensin-converting enzyme (ACE) inhibitor (telmisartan)

Contraindications

- Pregnancy and lactation
- Bilateral renal artery stenosis; kidney failure
- History of angioedema

Side Effects

- Angioedema—can be severe and life-threatening
- Fetal injury during second and third trimester
- Lower incidence of cough

Nursing Implications

1. Monitor effect of medication on blood pressure (BP).
2. Assess for angioedema on initial administration—discontinue immediately if it occurs.
3. Monitor kidney function.
4. Review patient's medications—has an additive effect; dosages of the other antihypertensive drugs may require reduction.
5. Monitor potassium levels, especially when given with potassium supplements.
6. Avoid salt substitutes with increased amounts of potassium.

Important nursing implications — Serious/life-threatening implications

Most frequent side effects — Patient teaching

NITROGLYCERIN

Tunnel Rats Excavation, Inc.
"Bigger Is Better"
We need to blow this tunnel open and widen it for better access. Send up the nitroglycerin!
DANGER
Delivery routes:
· Transdermal
· PO
· SL
· IV
Quick or slow release, watch out for severe hypotension, tachycardia, dizziness, headache, and syncope.
Quick-onset nitro 2-5 minutes IV
Slow-onset nitro 10-30 minutes SL TD
QUICK
NTG = IV
Sublingual
Tabs (SL)
Translingual spray
Transdermal patch
Nitro ointments
Sustained-release capsules
SLOW

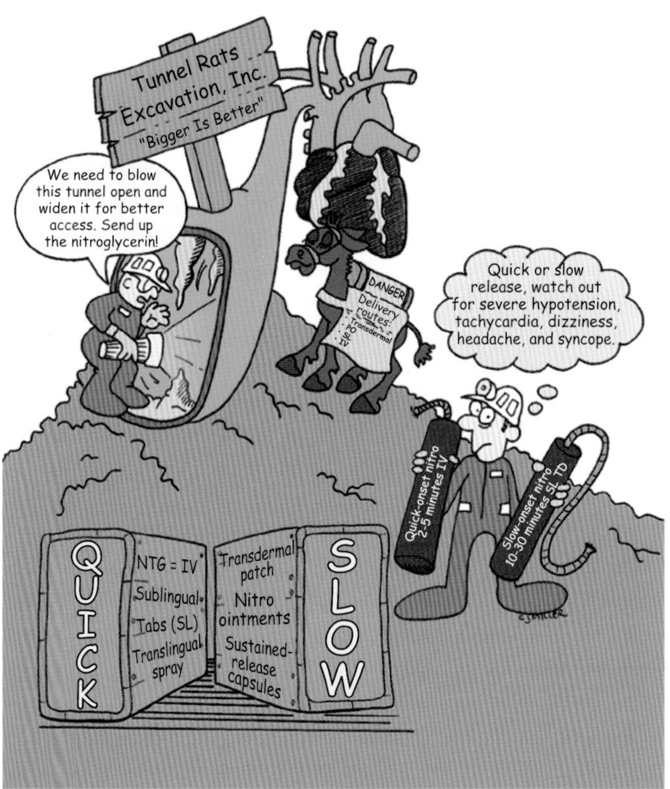

What You Need to Know

NITROGLYCERIN

Actions

Vasodilator that relaxes vascular smooth muscle (arterial and venous) system with more prominent effects on veins, which decreases preload. The modest arteriolar relaxation reduces systemic vascular resistance, which decreases afterload. These actions decrease cardiac oxygen demand.

Uses

- To relieve acute anginal pain and prevent further angina pain

Contraindications and Precautions

- Hypersensitive patients
- Severe anemia
- Erectile dysfunction medications (sildenafil [Viagra], tadalafil [Cialis], avanafil [Stendra], vardenafil [Levitra])
- Severe hepatic or renal disease and use of other vasodilators
- Beta-blockers, verapamil, diltiazem

Side Effects

- Orthostatic hypotension, headache, reflex tachycardia

Nursing Implications

1. Patients with angina should carry nitroglycerin with them at all times.
2. Teach proper storage for freshness (tingling, fizzle sensation under tongue). Discard unused medication after 24 months.
3. When angina occurs, teach patient to take a sublingual tablet (place under tongue); if pain is not relieved in 5 minutes, call 9-1-1. May take one tablet every 5 minutes for a total of 3 tablets while waiting for emergency care.
4. Avoid alcoholic beverages during nitroglycerin therapy.
5. Avoid swallowing or chewing sustained-release tablets to help drug reach gastrointestinal system.
6. Rotate transdermal patches and remove after 12 to 14 hours to have a "patch free" interval of 10 to 12 hours daily.
7. In hospitalized patients, check blood pressure (BP) before administering.
8. Teach to direct the translingual spray against the oral mucosa; warn patient not to inhale the spray.

Important nursing implications — Serious/life-threatening implications

Most frequent side effects — Patient teaching

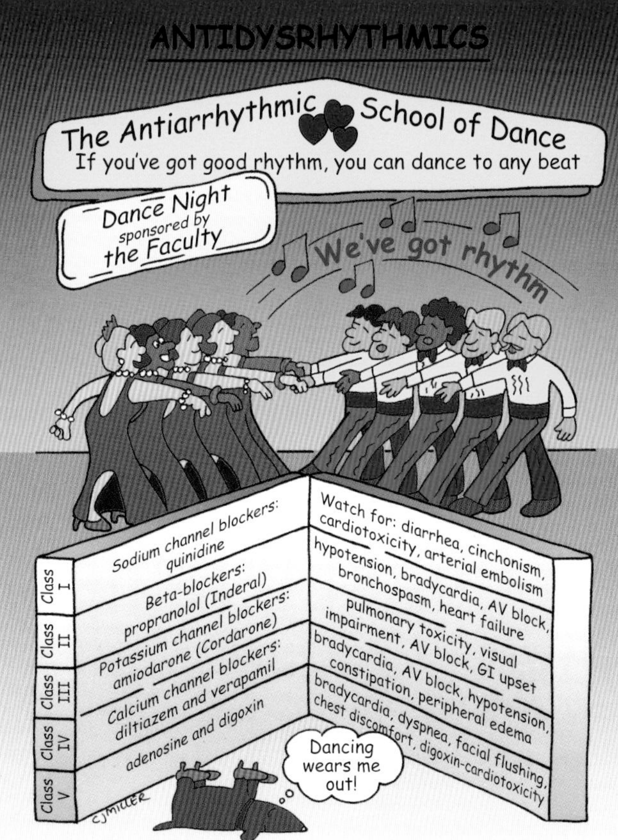
ANTIDYSRHYTHMICS
The Antiarrhythmic School of Dance
If you've got good rhythm, you can dance to any beat
Dance Night
sponsored by
the Faculty
We've got rhythm
Class I
Sodium channel blockers: quinidine
Watch for: diarrhea, cinchonism, cardiotoxicity, arterial embolism
Class II
Beta-blockers: propranolol (Inderal)
hypotension, bradycardia, AV block, bronchospasm, heart failure
Class III
Potassium channel blockers: amiodarone (Cordarone)
pulmonary toxicity, visual impairment, AV block, GI upset
Class IV
Calcium channel blockers: diltiazem and verapamil
bradycardia, AV block, hypotension, constipation, peripheral edema
Class V
adenosine and digoxin
bradycardia, dyspnea, facial flushing, chest discomfort, digoxin-cardiotoxicity
Dancing wears me out!
CJ MILLER

What You Need to Know

ANTIDYSRHYTHMICS

Actions

- *Sodium channel blockers* block sodium, slowing the impulse in the atria, ventricles, and nodal and Purkinje systems (quinidine, lidocaine).
- *Beta-adrenergic blockers* reduce automaticity in the sinoatrial (SA) node, slow conduction velocity in the atrioventricular (AV) node, reduce contractility in the atria and ventricles (Inderal), and prolong the PR interval.
- *Potassium channel blockers* delay repolarization of fast potentials, prolong action potential duration and effective refractory period (amiodarone), and prolong the QT interval.
- *Calcium channel blockers* block calcium channels and reduce the automaticity in the SA node, delay conduction through the AV node, delay reduction of myocardial contractility (diltiazem, verapamil), and prolong the PR interval.
- Adenosine and digoxin decrease conduction through the AV node and reduce automaticity of the SA node.

Uses

- Tachydysrhythmia: supraventricular tachycardia, paroxysmal atrial tachycardia, atrial fibrillation

Precaution

- Use with great caution in patients with AV block, bradycardia; medications can cause new dysrhythmias as well as exacerbate existing ones.

Side Effects

- Quinidine: cinchonism effects—tinnitus, headaches, nausea, vomiting, dizziness
- Hypotension, fatigue, bradycardia
- Amiodarone—pulmonary toxicity, visual impairment, cardiotoxicity, photosensitivity, thyroid toxicity (hypo- or hyperthyroidism), liver toxicity

Nursing Implications

1. Monitor cardiac rhythm, particularly during initial dose for effectiveness; report apical pulse rate less than 60 beats/min.
2. Report changes in dysrhythmias or occurrence of new one; assess for hypotension.
3. Instruct patient to take all prescribed doses and not to catch up on missed doses.
4. Instruct patient to report shortness of breath; pain; and irregular, fast, or slow heartbeats

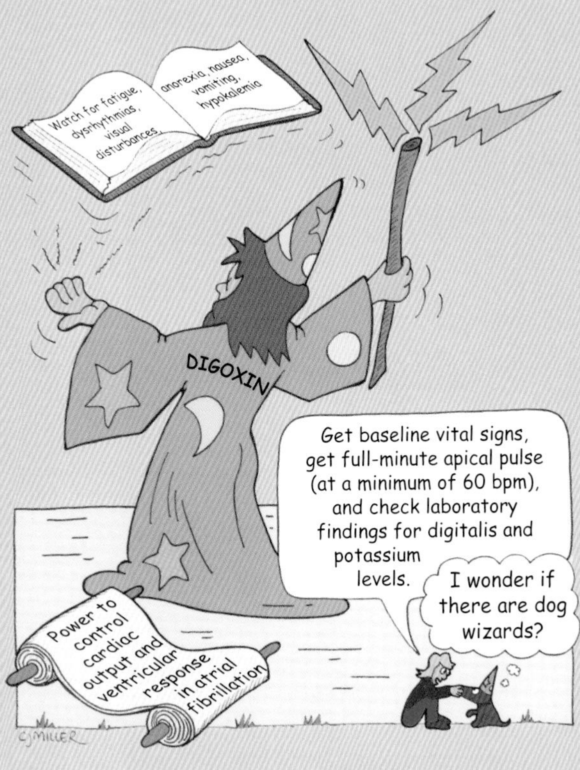
WIZARD OF DIGITALIS
Watch for fatigue, dysrhythmias, visual disturbances,
anorexia, nausea, vomiting, hypokalemia
DIGOXIN
Get baseline vital signs, get full-minute apical pulse (at a minimum of 60 bpm), and check laboratory findings for digitalis and potassium levels.
I wonder if there are dog wizards?
Power to control cardiac output and ventricular response in atrial fibrillation
CJMILLER

What You Need to Know

DIGITALIS

Actions

Affects the mechanical and electrical actions of the heart, which increases myocardial contractility (the force of ventricular contraction) and cardiac output. Alters the electrical activity in noncontractile tissue and ventricular muscle (e.g., automaticity, refractoriness, impulse conduction). Inhibits Na-K ATPase. Is classified as a cardiac glycoside.

Uses

- Heart failure—to improve cardiac output
- Atrial fibrillation and flutter

Contraindications and Precautions

- Hypersensitivity, ventricular tachycardia, ventricular fibrillation
- Renal insufficiency, hypokalemia, advanced heart failure, partial atrioventricular block, pregnancy
- When given with amiodarone, can increase digoxin level

Side Effects

- Dizziness, headache, malaise, fatigue
- Nausea, vomiting, visual disturbances (blurred or yellow vision; halos around dark objects), anorexia—frequently foreshadow serious toxicity
- Hypokalemia (most common reason for digoxin-related dysrhythmias is diuretic-induced hypokalemia), dysrhythmias, bradycardia

Nursing Implications

1. Monitor digoxin serum levels; check for toxicity (2 ng/mL is considered toxic). Digoxin has a narrow therapeutic range.
2. Monitor pulse, and teach patients to take their pulse. Report a pulse rate less than 60 or greater than 100 beats/min for adults and rates less than 100 beats/min for pediatric patients: hold the dose and notify a primary health care provider.
3. Administer intravenous (IV) doses slowly over 5 minutes.
4. Teach patients to not double up with missed doses.
5. Teach patients to recognize early signs of hypokalemia (muscle weakness) and digitalis toxicity (nausea, vomiting, anorexia, diarrhea, blurred or yellow visual disturbances, halos around dark objects), and notify health care provider.

Important nursing implications | Serious/life-threatening implications
Most frequent side effects | Patient teaching

LIDOCAINE TOXICITY

S – Slurred or difficult speech
- Paresthesias
- Numbness of lips/tongue

A – Altered cardiovascular system
- Drowsiness
- Dizziness
- Dysrhythmias
- Restlessness
- Hypotension
- Bradycardia, heart block

M – Muscle twitching
- Tremors

S – Seizures
- Respiratory depression
- Respiratory and cardiac arrest

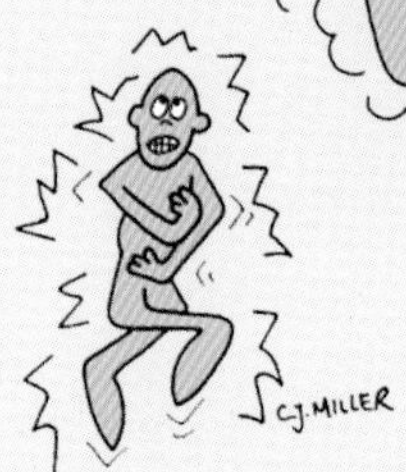

What You Need to Know

LIDOCAINE TOXICITY

Pathophysiology

Lidocaine is rapidly metabolized by the liver. If administered orally, the dose would be inactivated on the first pass through the liver. It is therefore given by intravenous (IV) infusion. Plasma drug levels are easily controlled. Its therapeutic range is 1.5 to 5.0 mcg/mL. In higher doses and at toxic levels, the central nervous and respiratory systems will be affected.

Effects on Heart and Electrocardiogram (ECG)

- Blocks sodium channels and slows conduction in atria and ventricles
- Reduces automaticity in ventricles and bundle of His–Purkinje system
- Accelerates repolarization
- No significant impact on ECG

Signs and Symptoms of Toxicity

- High and prolonged doses—drowsiness, confusion, paresthesias
- Toxic doses—seizure, respiratory arrest

Treatment

- Equipment for resuscitation (crash cart)
- Diazepam or phenytoin to be used for seizures

Nursing Implications

1. Assess level of consciousness and orientation.
2. Administer at prescribed IV rate—administration that is too rapid can cause problems.
3. Protect for possible seizure activity; assess for paresthesia.
4. Check vital signs frequently.
5. Monitor ECG and report unusual activity or changes in rhythm.
6. Assess respiratory system, ventilation, and gas exchange (oxygen saturation).
7. Lidocaine preparations that contain epinephrine must never be administered IV; doing so can cause severe hypertension and life-threatening dysrhythmias. Lidocaine used for local anesthesia often contains epinephrine.

Important nursing implications	Serious/life-threatening implications
Most frequent side effects	Patient teaching

DRUGS FOR BRADYCARDIA AND DECREASED BLOOD PRESSURE

= IDEA

I — SOPROTERENOL

D — OPAMINE

E — PINEPHRINE

A — TROPINE

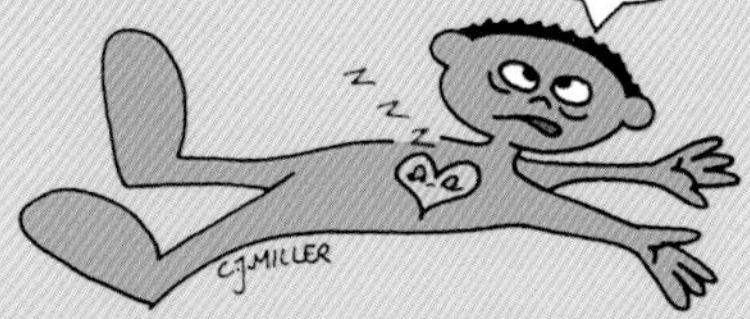

What You Need to Know

Drugs for Bradycardia and Decreased Blood Pressure

ISOPROTERENOL (ISUPREL)

Classification
Sympathomimetic, catecholamine

Actions
Increases heart rate and cardiac output, causes bronchodilation

Adverse Effects
Tachycardia and angina; can cause hyperglycemia in patients with diabetes

DOPAMINE

Classification
Sympathomimetic, catecholamine

Actions
At low doses, causes renal vasodilation. Moderate doses increase cardiac contractility, stroke volume, and cardiac output. Higher doses increase peripheral vascular resistance, blood pressure, and renal vasoconstriction.

Adverse Effects
Tachycardia, dysrhythmias, anginal pain, vasoconstriction leading to tissue necrosis with extravasation

EPINEPHRINE (ADRENALIN)

Classification
Adrenergic agonist, catecholamine

Actions
Causes vasoconstriction and increases heart rate; bronchodilator; treatment of choice for anaphylactic reactions

Adverse Effects
Hypertension, dysrhythmias, anginal pain, restlessness, necrosis following extravasation, hyperglycemia in patients with diabetes

ATROPINE

Classification
Anticholinergic, antidysrhythmic

Actions
Acts on smooth muscle of the heart and increases cardiac rate

Adverse Effects
Tachycardia, palpitations, dry mouth (xerostomia), drowsiness, blurred vision,

ALPHA-ADRENERGIC ANTAGONISTS (ALPHA-BLOCKERS) SIDE EFFECTS

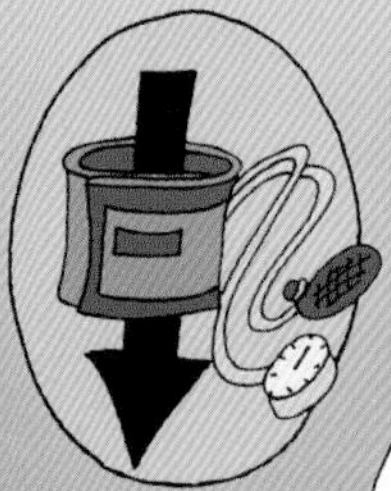

Orthostatic Hypotension

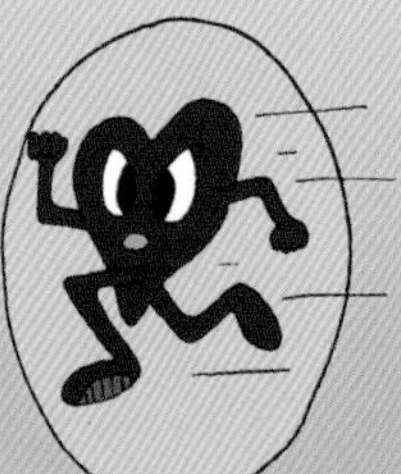

Reflex Tachycardia

Examples:

doxazosin (Cardura)
prazosin (Minipress)

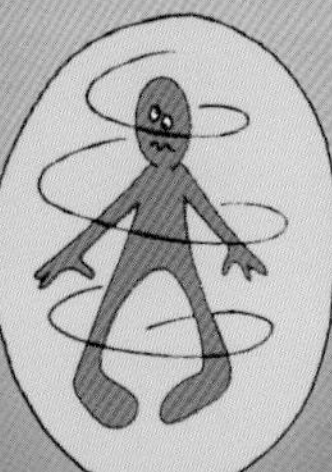

Dizziness

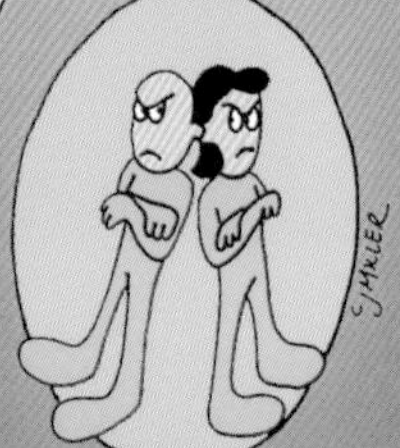

Sexual Dysfunction (inhibition of ejaculation)

What You Need to Know

ALPHA-ADRENERGIC ANTAGONISTS (ALPHA-BLOCKERS) SIDE EFFECTS

Examples

Doxazosin (Cardura), prazosin (Minipress), terazosin (Hytrin)

Actions

Stimulate central alpha-receptors, which decreases sympathetic outflow from the central nervous system, causing a decrease in peripheral vascular resistance and a slight decrease in cardiac output

Uses

- Mild-to-moderate hypertension

Precautions and Contraindications

- Hypersensitivity to drug and sulfites
- Patients with liver disease, blood dyscrasias, and pheochromocytoma

Side Effects

- Orthostatic hypotension
- Reflex tachycardia, dizziness, drowsiness, sedation
- Inhibition of ejaculation, nasal congestion, dry mouth

Nursing Implications

1. Watch for orthostatic hypotension, which is intensified with prolonged standing, hot baths or showers, hot weather, alcohol use, and strenuous exercise.
2. Patient should consume no more than 4 cups of caffeinated coffee, tea, or cola per day.
3. Patient should take medicine at bedtime to avoid drowsiness during the day.
4. Discontinue slowly to avoid rebound hypertension.
5. Teach patient about first-dose effect of severe orthostatic hypotension and to avoid hazardous activities and driving for 12 to 24 hours after initial dose. To decrease risk, instruct patient to take first dose at bedtime.

Important nursing implications | Serious/life-threatening implications

Most frequent side effects | Patient teaching

BETA-ADRENERGIC ANTAGONISTS (BETA-BLOCKERS) SIDE EFFECTS

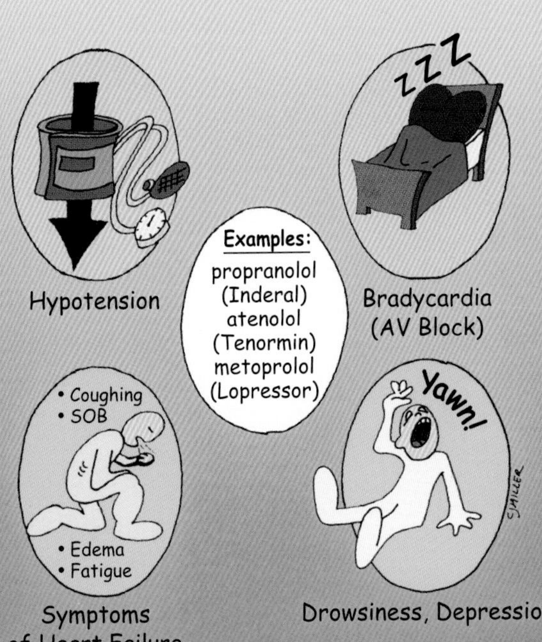

Symptoms of Heart Failure

Drowsiness, Depression

What You Need to Know

BETA-ADRENERGIC ANTAGONISTS (BETA-BLOCKERS) SIDE EFFECTS

Examples

Propranolol (Inderal), atenolol (Tenormin), metoprolol (Lopressor), nadolol (Corgard)

Actions

Block sympathetic nervous system catecholamines, resulting in reduced renin and aldosterone release and fluid balance. Vasodilation of arterioles leads to a decrease in pulmonary vascular resistance and blood pressure. Blockade leads to reduced heart rate, reduced force of contraction, and reduced velocity of impulse conduction through the atrioventricular (AV) node.

Uses

- Hypertension, antianginal agents in long-term treatment of angina
- Dysrhythmias—to suppress sinus and atrial tachydysrhythmias
- Myocardial infarction (MI), hyperthyroidism, migraine prophylaxis, pheochromocytoma, glaucoma

Contraindications

- AV block (if greater than first degree), bradydysrhythmias, severe allergies

Precautions

- Can cause bronchoconstriction; use with caution in patients with diabetes (masks signs of hypoglycemia), renal or hepatic dysfunction.
- History of depression

Side Effects

- Postural hypotension, bradycardia, drowsiness, depression, heart failure
- Bronchospasm, bronchoconstriction, malaise, lethargy

Nursing Implications

1. Assess vital signs; monitor closely if given with a calcium channel blocker.
2. Report any weakness, dizziness, bradycardia, or fainting.
3. Report any edema or difficulty breathing.
4. Monitor patients with diabetes; increased risk of hypoglycemia—tachycardia (a symptom of hypoglycemia) is often masked because of the $beta_1$ blockade.

Important nursing implications | Serious/life-threatening implications
Most frequent side effects | Patient teaching

HMG-CoA REDUCTASE INHIBITORS (Antihyperlipidemics)

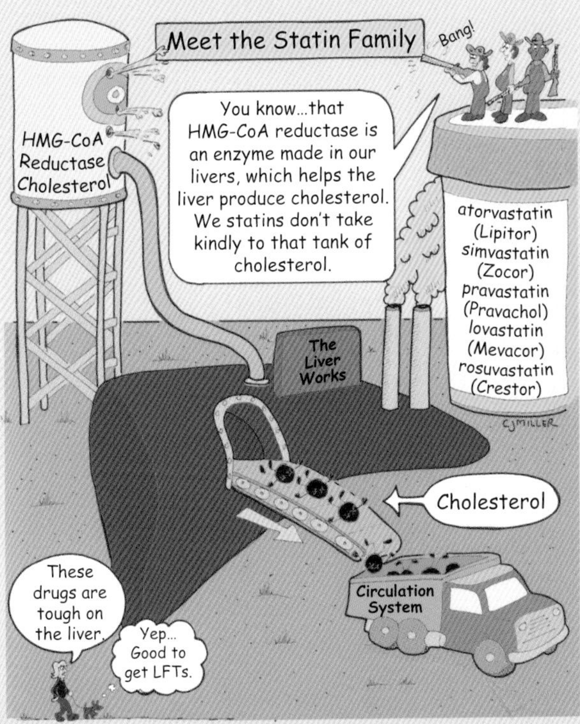

What You Need to Know

HMG-COA REDUCTASE INHIBITORS (STATINS)

Examples

Atorvastatin (Lipitor), simvastatin (Zocor), pravastatin (Pravachol), lovastatin (Mevacor), rosuvastatin (Crestor)

Action

Lower cholesterol levels by inhibiting the formation of HMG-CoA reductase, which is an enzyme that is required for the liver to synthesize cholesterol. Effective in decreasing low-density lipoprotein (LDL) and increasing high-density lipoprotein (HDL) levels and may lower triglycerides in some patients.

Uses

- Hypercholesterolemia
- Primary and secondary prevention of cardiovascular events
- Patients with type 2 diabetes and coronary heart disease

Contraindications

- Viral or alcoholic hepatitis; pregnancy (categorized as FDA category X)

Precautions

- Liver disease, depending on severity
- Excessive alcohol use

Side Effects

- Headache, rash, or gastrointestinal (GI) disturbances (dyspepsia, cramps, flatulence, constipation, abdominal pain)
- Myopathy—myositis, rhabdomyolysis (severe form; rarely occurs)
- Hepatotoxicity—liver injury with increases in levels of serum transaminases

Nursing Implications

1. Instruct patient to report unexplained muscle pain or tenderness.
2. Monitor liver function studies.
3. Inform women of childbearing age about the potential for fetal harm should they become pregnant.
4. Administer medication in the evening without regard to meals, except for lovastatin, which is taken with the evening meal (extended-release tablet taken at bedtime).
5. Instruct patient about dietary changes to reduce weight and cholesterol.

Important nursing implications | Serious/life-threatening implications

Most frequent side effects | Patient teaching

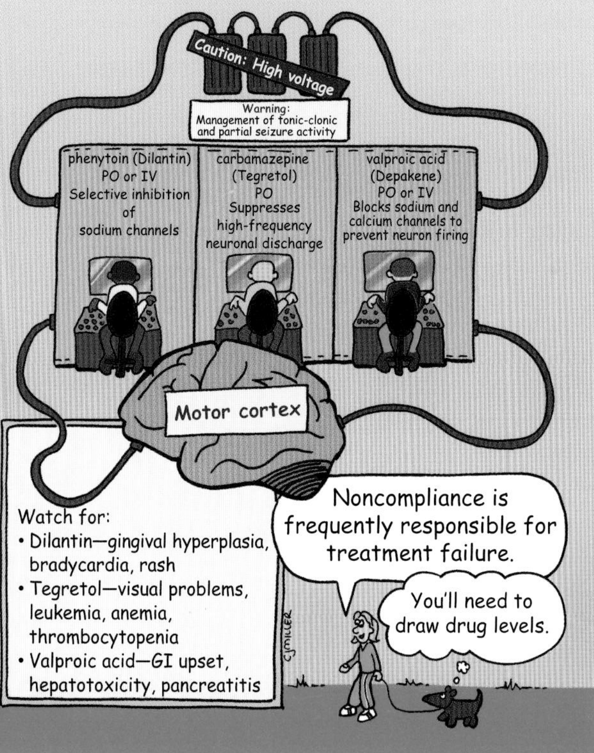
ANTIEPILEPTIC DRUGS
Caution: High voltage
Warning:
Management of tonic-clonic and partial seizure activity
phenytoin (Dilantin)
PO or IV
Selective inhibition of sodium channels
carbamazepine
(Tegretol)
PO
Suppresses high-frequency neuronal discharge
valproic acid
(Depakene)
PO or IV
Blocks sodium and calcium channels to prevent neuron firing
Motor cortex
Watch for:
• Dilantin—gingival hyperplasia, bradycardia, rash
• Tegretol—visual problems, leukemia, anemia, thrombocytopenia
• Valproic acid—GI upset, hepatotoxicity, pancreatitis
Noncompliance is frequently responsible for treatment failure.
You'll need to draw drug levels.
CJMILLER

What You Need to Know

ANTIEPILEPTIC DRUGS

Actions

Suppresses discharge of neurons within a seizure focus area and decreases spread of seizure activity to other areas of the brain

Uses

- Medications are specific to type of seizure (generalized or partial) and to specific categories of seizures.
- Can be used for status epilepticus.

Contraindications

- Hypersensitivity
- Pregnancy (teratogenic effects)

Precautions

- Hepatic, hematologic, and respiratory disorders
- Sinus bradycardia, sinoatrial block, second- and third-degree block (Dilantin)

Side Effects

- Valproic acid (Depakote): constipation, nausea, vomiting, hepatotoxicity, fatal pancreatitis
- Carbamazepine (Tegretol): blood dyscrasias, visual disturbances, ataxia, vertigo
- Phenytoin (Dilantin): nystagmus, cognitive impairment, hypotension, gingival hyperplasia, measles-like rash, ataxia

Nursing Implications

1. Usually given orally. Do not mix intravenous (IV) Dilantin with other medications. Give IV Dilantin slowly (do not exceed 50 mg/min).
2. Perform periodic blood studies for therapeutic levels.
3. Check hepatic and renal functions.
4. Teach patient to purchase a Medic-Alert bracelet or carry a medical ID card.
5. Teach patient to never abruptly discontinue medication.
6. With Dilantin, watch for gingival hyperplasia; encourage routine prophylactic dental care, and instruct patient to take with meals; suggest taking 0.5 mg of folic acid daily.
7. Do not give Tegretol with grapefruit juice.
8. Teach patient to report rash (Dilantin), signs of infection (Tegretol), signs of pancreatitis or liver injury (Valproic acid).

Important nursing implications   Serious/life-threatening implications

PROMETHAZINE (PHENERGAN)

Should have had Phenergan on board
Oh no! Not now!!!
Phenergan is used for motion sickness, vertigo, nausea and vomiting postoperatively and from chemotherapy
Captain
Phenergan
CJMILLER

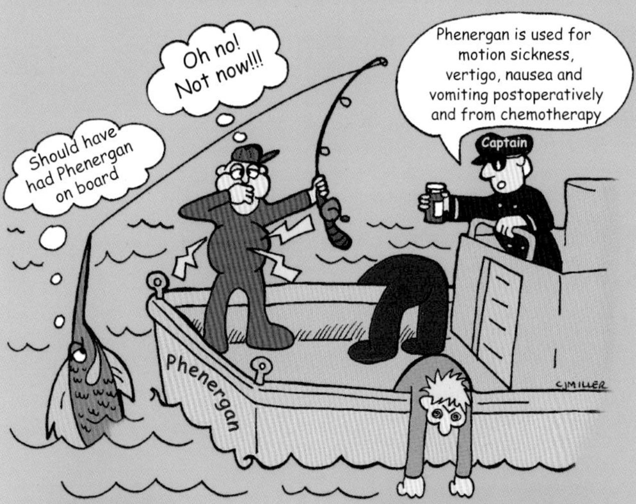

Delivery

PO
PR
IM
IV

Watch for:

- Drowsiness
- Restlessness
- Hypotension
- Confusion
- Urinary retention

What You Need to Know

PROMETHAZINE (PHENERGAN)

Classification

Antiemetic; antihistamine

Action

Blocks histamine receptors in the neuronal pathway, leading from the vestibular apparatus of the inner ear to the vomiting center in the medulla

Uses

- Nausea and vomiting

Contraindications and Precautions

- Children less than 2 years old contraindicated, and use with caution in children more than 2 years old—severe respiratory depression ■ Black Box Alert
- Glaucoma, gastrointestinal or genitourinary obstruction
- Pregnancy, seizures, asthma, severe central nervous system (CNS) depression

Side Effects

- Sedation, drowsiness, disorientation
- Hypotension, syncope in the older adult
- Severe respiratory depression, especially in children
- Dry mouth, urinary retention
- Epigastric distress, flushing, visual and hearing disturbances

Nursing Implications

1. Evaluate patient's respiratory status during use of this drug.
2. Teach patient to avoid tasks that require mental alertness; do not drink alcohol.
3. Direct patient to report tremors or abnormal body movements.
4. Long-term therapy: teach patient to have complete blood count (CBC) drawn.
5. If administered IV and extravasation occurs, severe tissue injury and necrosis can lead to amputation of extremity, so IM route is preferred.
6. Evaluate older adult's ability to urinate.

Important nursing implications | Serious/life-threatening implications
Most frequent side effects | Patient teaching

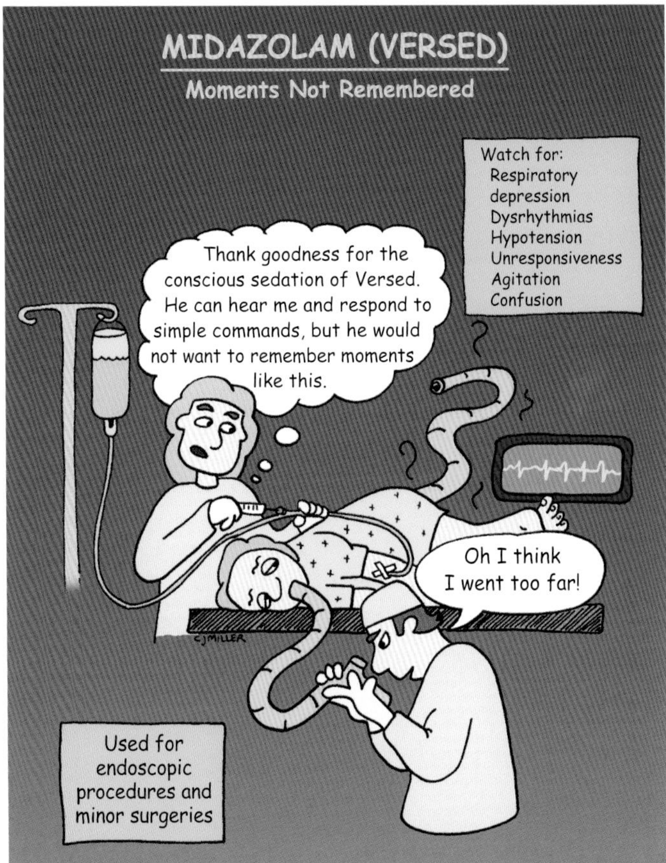

MIDAZOLAM (VERSED)
Moments Not Remembered
Watch for:
Respiratory depression
Dysrhythmias
Hypotension
Unresponsiveness
Agitation
Confusion
Thank goodness for the conscious sedation of Versed. He can hear me and respond to simple commands, but he would not want to remember moments like this.
Oh I think I went too far!
CJMILLER
Used for endoscopic procedures and minor surgeries

What You Need to Know

MIDAZOLAM (VERSED)

Classification

Benzodiazepine

Other benzodiazepines administered for induction of anesthesia—diazepam, lorazepam

Action

Produces unconsciousness and amnesia

Uses

- Induction of anesthesia and conscious sedation

Contraindications

- Shock, coma, acute alcohol intoxication, acute narrow-angle glaucoma

Precautions

- Can cause dangerous cardiorespiratory effects, including respiratory depression and cardiac arrest ■ Black Box Alert
- Acute illness, severe electrolyte imbalance
- Increased sedation effects with ingestion of grapefruit juice

Side Effects

- Decreased respiratory rate, tenderness at intramuscular/intravenous (IM/IV) injection site, hypotension

Nursing Implications

1. Administer slowly over 2 or more minutes. Wait another 2 or more minutes for full effects to develop before giving additional doses to avoid cardiorespiratory problems.
2. Unconsciousness develops quickly (within 60 to 80 seconds). Conscious sedation persists for approximately 1 hour.
3. Perform constant cardiac and respiratory monitoring during administration with resuscitative equipment nearby.
4. The patient will not remember any postoperative instructions. After outpatient procedures, the patient must be accompanied home by a responsible adult.
5. The patient should not operate a car or engage in activities requiring alertness for 24 hours after receiving medication.

Important nursing implications | Serious/life-threatening implications

Most frequent side effects | Patient teaching

BENZODIAZEPINE-LIKE DRUGS

When the Day Keeps You Awake at Night

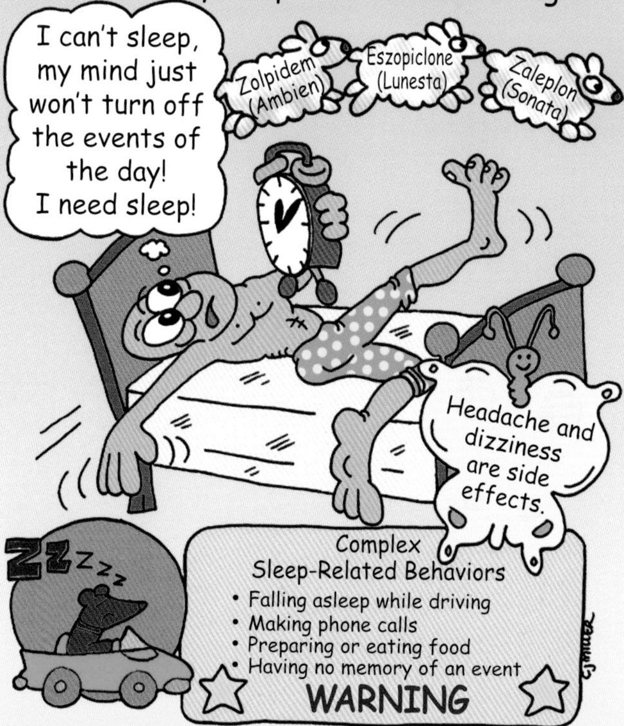

What You Need to Know

BENZODIAZEPINE-LIKE DRUGS

Action

Act as agonist at the benzodiazepine receptor site on the gamma-aminobutyric acid (GABA) receptor

Uses

- Insomnia
    - Zolpidem (Ambien) and zaleplon (Sonata)—short-term treatment for insomnia
    - Eszopiclone (Lunesta)—no limitation on length of usage

Contraindications and Precautions

- Pregnancy, lactation
- Hepatic impairment, depression, history of drug usage

Side Effects

- Drowsiness, dizziness, confusion
- Bitter aftertaste (eszopiclone)
- Sleep-related complex behaviors—sleep driving, making phone calls, preparing food while asleep, and having no memory of the activity

Nursing Implications

1. Is a Schedule IV substance—low potential for tolerance, dependence, or abuse.
2. Can intensify effects of other hypnotics.
3. Teach patient to not break or chew the extended-release capsules.
4. Teach patient to not use medication in combination with alcohol.
5. Encourage patient to take the medication immediately before going to bed—do not participate in activities that require mental alertness.
6. Teach patient measures to enhance sleep—decreased consumption of caffeine-containing beverages (e.g., coffee, tea, colas), warm milk, bathing, quiet environment, reading, comfort measures.
7. Carefully assess effects on older adult patients.

Important nursing implications	Serious/life-threatening implications
Most frequent side effects	Patient teaching

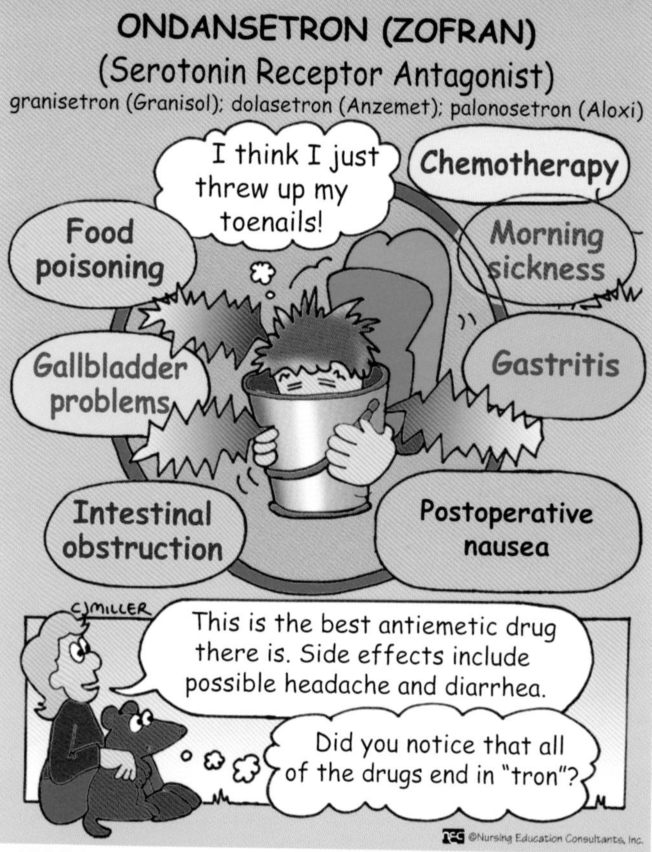
ONDANSETRON (ZOFRAN)
(Serotonin Receptor Antagonist)
granisetron (Granisol); dolasetron (Anzemet); palonosetron (Aloxi)
I think I just threw up my toenails!
Chemotherapy
Food poisoning
Morning sickness
Gallbladder problems
Gastritis
Intestinal obstruction
Postoperative nausea
CJMILLER
This is the best antiemetic drug there is. Side effects include possible headache and diarrhea.
Did you notice that all of the drugs end in "tron"?
©Nursing Education Consultants, Inc.

What You Need to Know

ONDANSETRON (ZOFRAN)

Classification

Antiemetic (serotonin receptor antagonist)

Other serotonin receptor antagonists are granisetron (Granisol), dolasetron (Anzemet), and palonosetron (Aloxi).

Actions

Prevents nausea and vomiting by blocking type 3 serotonin receptors (5-HT receptors) located in the chemoreceptor trigger zone (CTZ) and on afferent vagal neurons in the upper gastrointestinal (GI) tract. Does not cause extrapyramidal effects (e.g., akathisia, acute dystonia) as seen with phenothiazide antiemetics.

Uses

- Chemotherapy-induced nausea and vomiting (CINV)
- Anesthesia
- Morning sickness of pregnancy
- Gastritis

Precautions

- Children and older adult patients
- Patients with long QT syndrome
- Electrolyte abnormalities, heart failure
- Bradydysrhythmias

Side Effects

- Headache, dizziness, drowsiness
- Diarrhea, constipation, abdominal pain
- Prolongs the QT interval (Zofran only) and poses a risk of torsades de pointes (life-threatening dysrhythmia)

Nursing Implications

1. Assess for effectiveness of medication—absence of nausea and vomiting during chemotherapy, anesthesia, gastritis, and morning sickness of pregnancy.
2. Monitor for side effects—anticipate patient requiring an analgesic (e.g., acetaminophen) for headache.
3. Teach patient to report diarrhea, constipation, rash, changes in respiration, or discomfort at the injection site.
4. Administer intravenous piggyback (IVPB) preparations slowly over 15 minutes.

Important nursing implications | Serious/life-threatening implications

Most frequent side effects | Patient teaching

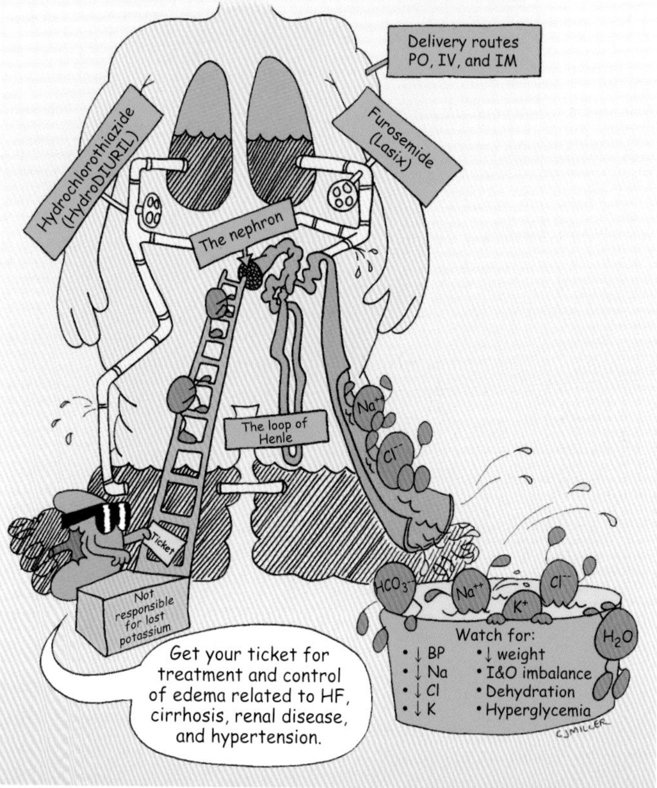
DIURETIC WATER SLIDE
Delivery routes
PO, IV, and IM
Hydrochlorothiazide
(HydroDIURIL)
Furosemide
(Lasix)
The nephron
The loop of
Henle
Na++
Cl--
Ticket
Not
responsible
for lost
potassium
Get your ticket for
treatment and control
of edema related to HF,
cirrhosis, renal disease,
and hypertension.
HCO3--
Na++
K+
Cl--
H2O
Watch for:
• ↓ BP
• ↓ Na
• ↓ Cl
• ↓ K
• ↓ weight
• I&O imbalance
• Dehydration
• Hyperglycemia
CJMILLER

What You Need to Know

DIURETICS

Actions

Loop diuretics inhibit sodium (Na) and chloride (Cl) reabsorption through direct action primarily in the ascending loop of Henle but also in the proximal and distal tubules. Thiazide diuretics act primarily on the distal convoluted tubule, inhibiting Na and Cl reabsorption.

Uses

- To treat edema that involves fluid volume excess resulting from a number of disorders of the heart, liver, or kidney
- Hypertension

Contraindications and Precautions

- Not recommended during pregnancy, breast-feeding
- Severe adrenocortical impairment
- Fluid and electrolyte depletion, gout
- Use with caution in patients taking digitalis, lithium, nonsteroidal antiinflammatory drugs (NSAIDs), and other antihypertensive medications

Side Effects

- Dehydration, hyponatremia, hypochloremia, hypokalemia
- Unusual tiredness, weakness, dizziness
- Irregular heartbeat, weak pulse, orthostatic hypotension
- Tinnitus, hyperglycemia, hyperuricemia, hearing loss (Lasix)

Nursing Implications

1. Monitor for adequate intake and output and potassium loss.
2. Monitor patient's weight and vital signs.
3. Monitor for signs and symptoms of hearing loss, which may last from 1 to 24 hours.
4. Teach patient to take medication early in the day to decrease nocturia.
5. Teach patient to report any hearing loss or signs of gout.

Important nursing implications	Serious/life-threatening implications
Most frequent side effects	Patient teaching

FUROSEMIDE (LASIX)

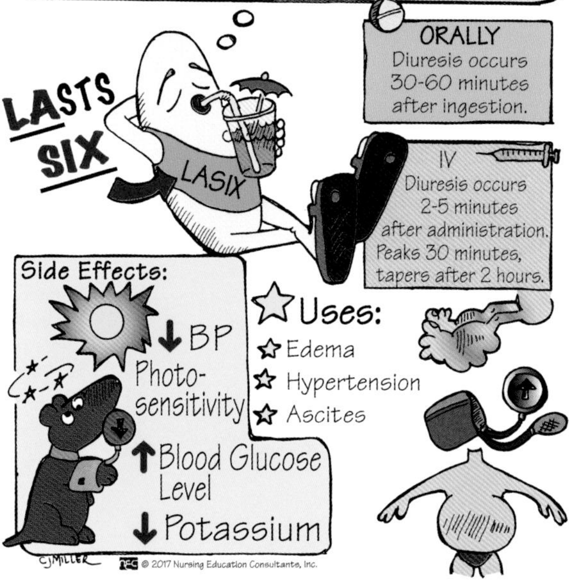

What You Need to Know

FUROSEMIDE (LASIX)

Actions

Furosemide inhibits sodium (Na) and chloride (Cl) reabsorption through direct action primarily in the ascending loop of Henle but also in the proximal and distal tubules. Also known as a "high-ceiling" diuretic.

Uses

- Pulmonary edema associated with heart failure (HF)
- Edema of hepatic, cardiac, or renal origin that has been unresponsive to less efficacious diuretics
- Hypertension that cannot be controlled with other diuretics

Contraindications and Precautions

- Not recommended during pregnancy (Category C), breast-feeding
- Severe adrenocortical impairment
- Fluid and electrolyte depletion, gout
- Use with caution in patients taking digitalis, ototoxic drugs, potassium-sparing diuretics, lithium, nonsteroidal antiinflammatory drugs (NSAIDs), and other antihypertensive medications

Side Effects

- Dehydration ■ Black Box Alert
- Hyponatremia, hypochloremia, hypokalemia
- Orthostatic hypotension (dizziness, lightheadedness, fainting)
- Hyperglycemia, hyperuricemia
- Transient hearing loss
- Reduces high-density lipoprotein (HDL) cholesterol and raises low-density lipoprotein (LDL) cholesterol and triglycerides
- Magnesium deficiency (hypomagnesemia)
- Increase urinary excretion of calcium leading to hypocalcemia

Nursing Implications

1. Monitor for adequate intake and output and potassium loss.
2. Monitor patient's weight and vital signs.
3. Monitor for signs and symptoms of hearing loss.
4. Teach patient to take medication early in the day to decrease nocturia.
5. Teach patient to report any hearing loss or signs of gout.

Important nursing implications	Serious/life-threatening implications
Most frequent side effects	Patient teaching

HYDROCHLOROTHIAZIDE

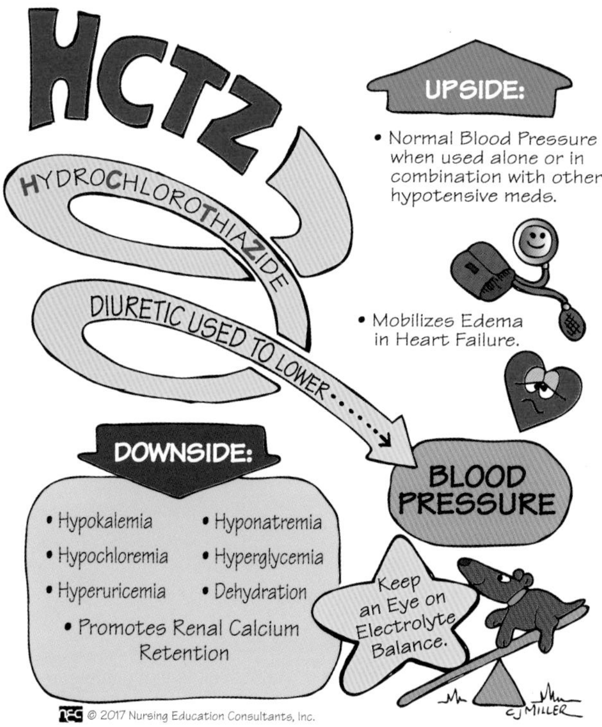

What You Need to Know

HYDROCHLOROTHIAZIDE (HCTZ)

Actions

Hydrochlorothiazide (HCTZ) promotes urine production by blocking the reabsorption of sodium (Na) and chloride (Cl) in the early segment of the distal convoluted tubule.

Uses

- Essential hypertension
- Edema of hepatic, cardiac, or renal origin
- Diabetes insipidus—reduce urine production by 30% to 50%; not clear on mechanism of this paradoxical effect
- Protection against postmenopausal osteoporosis by promoting tubular reabsorption of calcium

Contraindications and Precautions

- Not recommended during pregnancy (Category C), breast-feeding
- Severe adrenocortical impairment
- Fluid and electrolyte depletion, gout
- Use with caution in patients taking digitalis, ototoxic drugs, potassium-sparing diuretics, lithium, nonsteroidal antiinflammatory drugs (NSAIDs), and other antihypertensive medications

Side Effects

- Hyponatremia, hypochloremia, hypokalemia, dehydration
- Orthostatic hypotension (dizziness, lightheadedness, fainting)
- Hyperglycemia, hyperuricemia
- Increases low-density lipoprotein (LDL) cholesterol, total cholesterol, and triglycerides
- Magnesium deficiency (hypomagnesemia)

Nursing Implications

1. Monitor for adequate intake and output and potassium loss.
2. Monitor patient's weight and vital signs.
3. Monitor for signs and symptoms of hearing loss.
4. Teach patient to take medication early in the day to decrease nocturia.
5. Teach patient to take medication with or after meals if gastrointestinal (GI) upset occurs.
6. Teach patient to report any signs of gout.

Important nursing implications   Serious/life-threatening implications

SPIRONOLACTONE
(Aldactone)

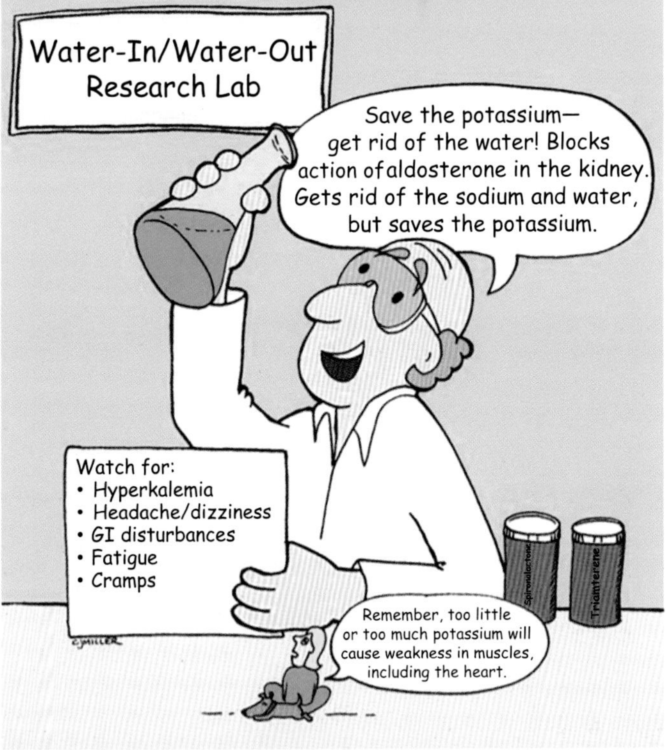

Water-In/Water-Out
Research Lab

Save the potassium—
get rid of the water! Blocks
action of aldosterone in the kidney.
Gets rid of the sodium and water,
but saves the potassium.

Watch for:
- Hyperkalemia
- Headache/dizziness
- GI disturbances
- Fatigue
- Cramps

Remember, too little
or too much potassium will
cause weakness in muscles,
including the heart.

Spironolactone

Triamterene

What You Need to Know

SPIRONOLACTONE (ALDACTONE)

Classification

Potassium-sparing diuretic

Actions

Blocks the action of aldosterone in the distal nephron, which leads to retention of potassium and increased excretion of sodium. Effects of spironolactone are delayed, taking up to 48 hours to develop, so action is not immediate.

Uses

- Treats hypertension and edema
- Reduces edema in patients with severe heart failure
- Primary hyperaldosteronism, premenstrual syndrome, polycystic ovary syndrome, acne in young women

Contraindications

- Hypersensitivity or renal failure
- Anuria
- Hyperkalemia

Precautions

- Renal and hepatic dysfunction

Side Effects

- Hyperkalemia
- Weakness, gastrointestinal (GI) disturbances, and leg cramps
- Dehydration
- Endocrine effects: hirsutism, menstrual irregularities, gynecomastia, impotence, deepening of voice

Nursing Implications

1. Monitor intake and output, and watch for cardiac dysrhythmias.
2. Monitor levels of electrolytes (e.g., potassium, sodium); do not administer with potassium supplements or salt substitutes containing potassium chloride.
3. Teach patient to report leg cramps, weakness, fatigue, or nausea.
4. Teach patient to restrict intake of potassium-rich foods (e.g., nuts, dried fruits, spinach, citrus fruits, potatoes, bananas).
5. Teach patient to take medication with or after meals if GI upset occurs.
6. Have patient notify health care provider if menstrual irregularities, gynecomastia, or impotence occurs.

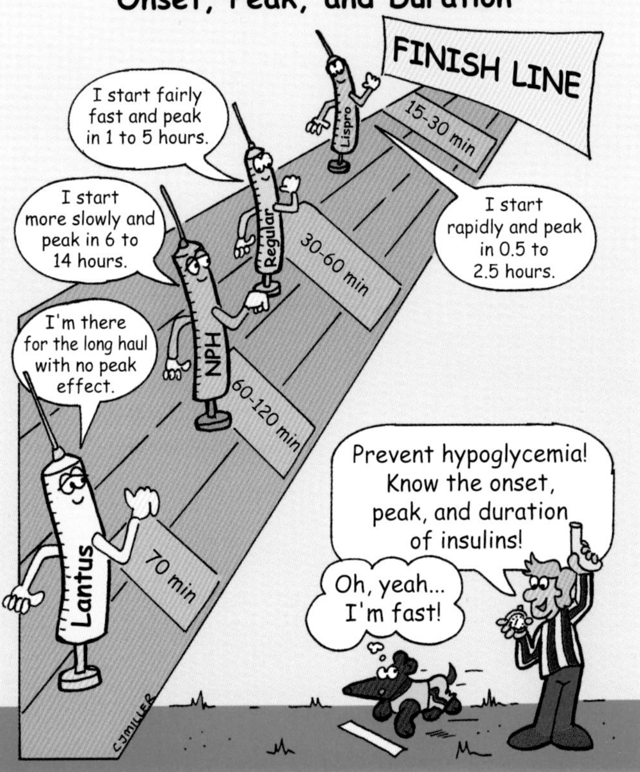
TYPES OF INSULIN
Onset, Peak, and Duration
FINISH LINE
I start fairly fast and peak in 1 to 5 hours.
I start more slowly and peak in 6 to 14 hours.
I'm there for the long haul with no peak effect.
I start rapidly and peak in 0.5 to 2.5 hours.
Lispro
Regular
NPH
Lantus
15-30 min
30-60 min
60-120 min
70 min
Prevent hypoglycemia! Know the onset, peak, and duration of insulins!
Oh, yeah... I'm fast!
CJMILLER

What You Need to Know

TYPES OF INSULIN

Actions ▲ High Alert

	Onset (min)	Peak (hr)	Duration (hr)
Short Duration: Rapid Acting			
Insulin lispro (Humalog)	15-30	0.5-2.5	3-6
Insulin aspart (NovoLog)	10-20	1-3	3-5
Insulin glulisine (Apidra)	10-15	1-1.5	3-5
Short Duration: Slow Acting			
Regular insulin (Humulin R, Novolin R)	30-60	1-5	6-10
Intermediate Duration			
NPH insulin (Humulin N, Novolin N)	60-120	6-14	16-24
Long Duration			
Insulin glargine (Lantus)	70	None	18-24
Insulin detemir (Levemir)	60-120	12-24	Varies

From Burchum JR, Rosenthal LD: *Lehne's pharmacology for nursing care*, ed 9, St Louis, 2016, Elsevier.

Nursing Implications

1. U100 insulin is the most common concentration.
2. NPH is the only cloudy insulin; roll vial gently between palms to mix.
3. Draw up clear (regular, lispro, aspart, and glulisine—short acting) before the cloudy (intermediate, NPH) insulin to prevent contaminating a short-acting insulin with a long-acting insulin.
4. Inject subcutaneously; aspiration is not necessary.
5. Avoid massaging the site after injection.
6. Rotate sites within anatomic area; the abdomen is preferred for more rapid, even absorption.
7. Only NPH (Humulin) can be mixed with short-acting insulins.
8. Only the short-acting insulins may be administered intravenously (IV).
9. Hypoglycemia is the primary drawback in maintaining tight control of glucose level.
10. Store unopened vials of insulin in the refrigerator; vial currently in use should be stored at room temperature for 1 month.
11. Prefilled syringes should be stored vertically with the needle pointing up to avoid clogging the needle; gently agitate the syringe to resuspend the insulin before use. May be stored in refrigerator for at least 1 week, perhaps 2 weeks.

ORAL ANTIDIABETIC DRUGS & NON-INSULIN INJECTABLE AGENTS

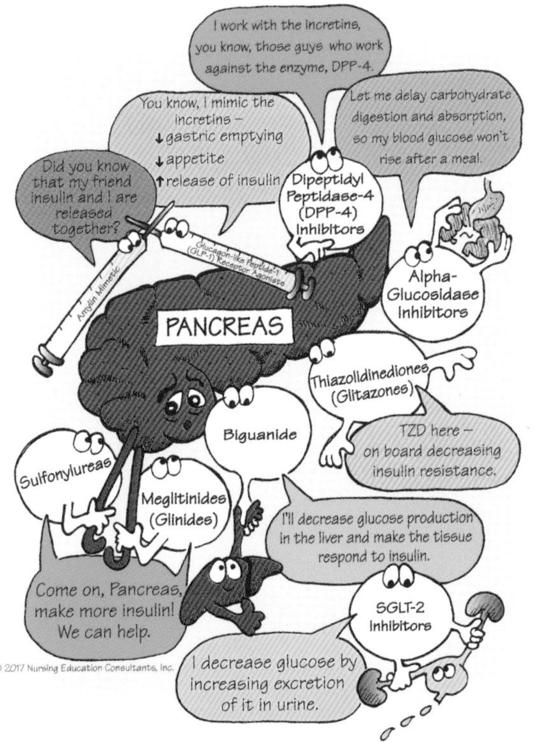

What You Need to Know

ORAL ANTIDIABETIC DRUGS AND NONINSULIN INJECTABLE AGENTS

Types

- Oral Antidiabetic Drugs
  - Seven types are available: the biguanides, sulfonylureas, meglitinides (glinides), thiazolidinediones (glitazones), alpha-glucosidase inhibitors, dipeptidyl peptidase-4 (DPP-4) inhibitors (gliptins), and sodium-glucose cotransporter 2 (SGLT-2) inhibitors.
  - Used for type 2 diabetes.
- Noninsulin Injectable Agents
  - Glucagon-like peptide-1 (GLP-1) receptor agonists: exenatide (Byetta), liraglutide (Victoza)
    - Indicated for only type 2 diabetes
  - Amylin mimetic: pramlintide (Symlin)
    - Can be used for type 1 and type 2 diabetes

Actions

- Sulfonylureas and meglitinides (glinides), collectively referred to as "insulin secretagogues," decrease blood glucose by increasing insulin release from beta cells of the pancreas.
- Metformin (a biguanide), the alpha-glucosidase inhibitors, and SGLT-2 inhibitors don't decrease blood glucose, but simply modulate the rise in glucose that happens after a meal.
- Thiazolidinediones (glitazones or TZDs) reduce insulin resistance and may decrease glucose production; only one medication is available, pioglitazone (Actos).
- Alpha-glucosidase inhibitors (acarbose, miglitol) act in the intestine to delay absorption of carbohydrates.
- DPP-4 inhibitors (gliptins) enhance the action of the incretin hormones, which stimulate glucose-dependent release of insulin and suppress postprandial release of glucagon (decreases glucose production in the liver).
- SGLT-2 inhibitors (flozins or gliflozins) block the reabsorption of filtered glucose in the kidney, leading to glucosuria.

Nursing Implications

1. Teach patient the symptoms of hypoglycemia (fatigue, hunger, cool moist skin, increased anxiety, dizziness, palpitations) that should be treated immediately by taking fast-acting oral carbohydrates (e.g., glucose tablets, orange juice).
2. Metformin—first-line drug therapy— is started immediately after the patient is diagnosed with type 2 diabetes

SULFONYLUREAS

Beta's Pancreatic Farms
The Best Beta Cells Around
• Monitor for hypoglycemia.
• Avoid during pregnancy and lactation.
• Avoid alcohol use.
Look at this girl produce insulin with just a little bit of stimulus.
CJMILLER
Glipizide
These drugs are indicated only for type 2 diabetes.
© 2016 Nursing Education Consultants, Inc.

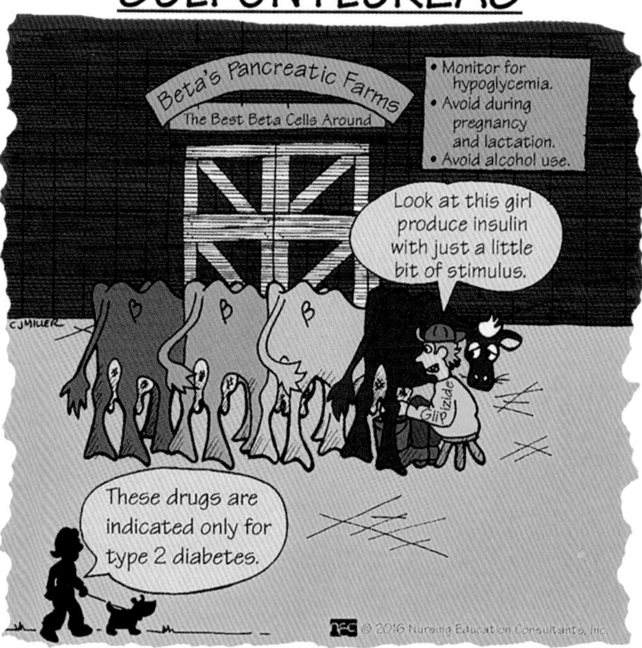

What You Need to Know

SULFONYLUREAS

- First generation*—tolbutamide (Orinase), chlorpropamide (generic only), tolazamide (generic only) ▲ High Alert
- Second generation—glipizide (Glucotrol), glyburide (DiaBeta), glimepiride (Amaryl)

Actions

Stimulates the beta cells of the pancreas to increase release of insulin. May also increase cellular sensitivity to insulin. Second-generation medications act the same but are stronger.

Uses

- Type 2 diabetes mellitus
- Used as adjunct to diet and exercise programs to maintain glucose control

Contraindications and Precautions

- Pregnancy and breast-feeding
- Not effective in patients with type 1 diabetes mellitus
- Use with caution in patients with adrenal or pituitary insufficiency or severe hepatic or renal impairment

Side Effects

- Hypoglycemia

Nursing Implications

1. Instruct patient to take with food if gastrointestinal (GI) upset occurs; otherwise, take the drug 15 to 30 minutes before meals. Do *not* take medication and skip meals.
2. Self-monitor blood glucose (SMBG) levels as directed.
3. Teach patient to maintain weight and dietary restrictions along with medication; avoid alcohol.
4. Hypoglycemia (fatigue, hunger, cool moist skin, increased anxiety, dizziness, palpitations) should be treated immediately—take fast-acting oral carbohydrates (e.g., glucose tablets, orange juice).
5. If patient is not in the hospital and cannot swallow, emergency services (9-1-1) should be initiated.

---

*First-generation agents used rarely.

METFORMIN (GLUCOPHAGE)

I'm Inspector Metformin. My team is here to help control blood glucose in type 2 diabetes.

FBG

HbA1c

Got to slow down glucose production in the liver.

Liver

Need to block the absorption of sugar in the intestines.

Intestines

Metformin helps the muscles use the sugar more efficiently.

Muscles

Dogs and cats can get diabetes. We need to "paws" for control.

Everyone is after a little sugar. Metformin can be used with other hypoglycemics.

Paws...I get it.

C.MILLER

What You Need to Know

METFORMIN (GLUCOPHAGE)

Classification

Oral antidiabetic ▲ High Alert

Actions

Lowers blood glucose and improves glucose tolerance by inhibiting glucose production in the liver, reducing (slightly) glucose absorption in the gut, and sensitizing insulin receptors at sites in fat and skeletal muscle

Uses

- Lowers blood glucose level in patients with type 2 diabetes
- May be used for blood glucose level control in patients with gestational diabetes
- Off-label use—polycystic ovary syndrome (PCOS)

Contraindications

- Conditions that predispose a patient to lactic acidosis (e.g., liver disease, severe infections, hypoxemia, dehydration), severe renal dysfunction

Precautions

- Patients who consume large amounts of alcohol
- Heart failure may predispose patient to lactic acidosis
- Patients with renal failure

Side Effects

- Decreased appetite, nausea, diarrhea
- Decreases absorption of vitamin B_{12} and folic acid

Nursing Implications

1. Monitor serum glucose and HbA_{1c} levels.
2. Assess effectiveness of blood glucose level control when used with other oral hypoglycemics (sulfonylureas).
3. Teach patient to:
    - Avoid alcohol.
    - Take medication as scheduled (do not skip or add doses; do not stop taking medication).
    - Maintain dietary restrictions for glucose control.
4. Teach patient the signs of lactic acidosis: hyperventilation, muscle aches, extreme fatigue.
5. Encourage increase in vitamin B_{12} and folic acid in diet.

Important nursing implications — Serious/life-threatening implications

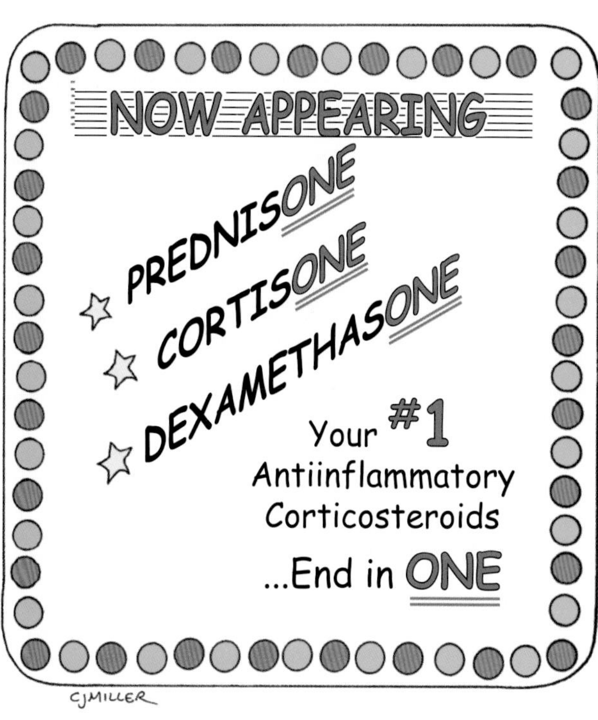
NOW APPEARING
PREDNISONE
CORTISONE
DEXAMETHASONE
Your #1
Antiinflammatory
Corticosteroids
...End in ONE
CJMILLER

What You Need to Know

CORTICOSTEROIDS

Classification

Adrenocorticosteroid, glucocorticoid

Actions

Suppress the inflammatory and immune systems by inhibiting synthesis of chemical mediators—prostaglandins, leukotrienes, and histamine. Decrease inflammation, which then reduces swelling, warmth, redness, and pain.

Uses

- Addison disease, hormone replacement therapy, cancer therapy
- To decrease inflammation—systemic lupus erythematosus, rheumatoid arthritis, inflammatory bowel disease, allergic conditions, asthma, chronic obstructive pulmonary disease, respiratory distress syndrome in infants
- To suppress graft rejection

Precautions

- Pediatric patients, pregnancy, and breast-feeding
- Hypertension, heart failure, renal impairment
- Esophagitis, peptic ulcer disease (PUD), and diabetes

Side Effects

- Increased risk of new infection, mask development of infection, and delayed wound healing
- Osteoporosis, glucose intolerance (hyperglycemia), peptic ulcer, gastrointestinal (GI) bleeding
- Muscle wasting, fluid and electrolyte disturbance, Cushing syndrome

Nursing Implications

1. Monitor fluid balance and potassium and glucose levels.
2. Warn patient to take as prescribed and not to discontinue therapy suddenly.
3. Assess for underlying infection and decreased wound healing.
4. Daily doses need to increase during stress.
5. Assess for Cushing symptoms.
6. Check stools for occult blood.
7. Advise patients to wear a Medic-Alert bracelet.
8. Teach about alternate-day dosing if ordered and taking medicine before 9 AM.

Important nursing implications | Serious/life-threatening implications

Most frequent side effects | Patient teaching

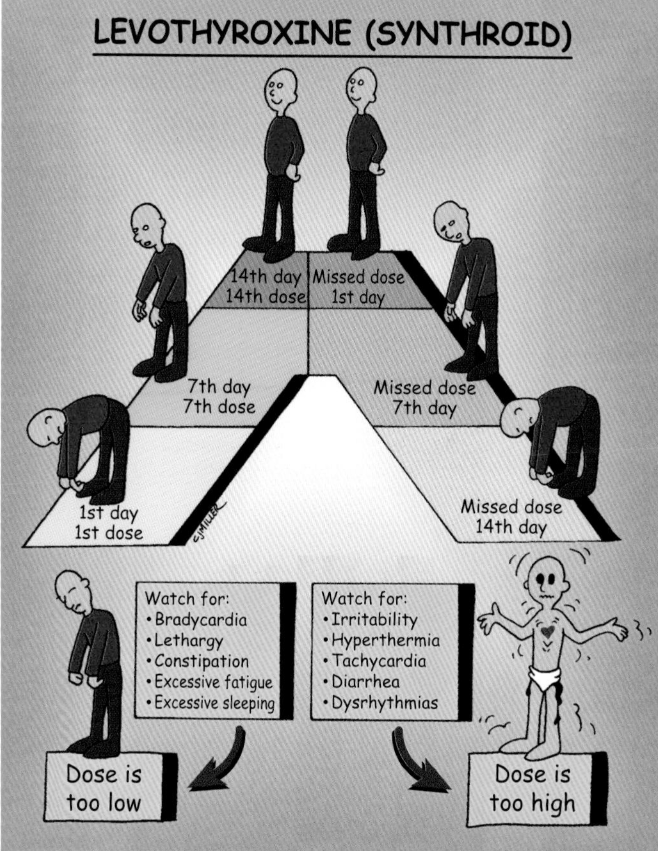
LEVOTHYROXINE (SYNTHROID)
14th day
14th dose
Missed dose
1st day
7th day
7th dose
Missed dose
7th day
1st day
1st dose
Missed dose
14th day
CJMILLER
Watch for:
• Bradycardia
• Lethargy
• Constipation
• Excessive fatigue
• Excessive sleeping
Watch for:
• Irritability
• Hyperthermia
• Tachycardia
• Diarrhea
• Dysrhythmias
Dose is too low
Dose is too high

What You Need to Know

LEVOTHYROXINE (SYNTHROID)

Classification

Thyroid hormone; synthetic preparation of thyroxine (T_4)

Actions

Increases basal metabolic rate, enhances gluconeogenesis, stimulates protein synthesis

Uses

- Replacement in decreased or absent thyroid function
- Hypothyroidism, cretinism, myxedema coma, simple goiter
- Management of thyroid cancer following surgery

Contraindications and Precautions

- Thyrotoxicosis and myocardial infarction without hypothyroidism
- Treatment of obesity
- Hypersensitivity
- Older adult patients, patients with impaired cardiac function, hypertension

Side Effects

- Overdose may cause thyrotoxicosis—tachycardia, increased blood pressure, angina, tremor, nervousness, insomnia, heat intolerance
- Long-term use—osteoporosis and increased risk for atrial fibrillation

Nursing Implications

1. Monitor for tachycardia and irregular pulse rate.
2. Teach patient to report any symptoms of thyrotoxicosis.
3. Replacement for hypothyroidism is lifelong. Do not discontinue.
4. Instruct patient to have thyroid-stimulating hormone levels measured periodically.
5. Takes approximately 6 to 8 weeks for the full effects of the medication to be seen.
6. Teach patient to take the medication in the morning, preferably 30 to 60 minutes before meals.

Important nursing implications
Serious/life-threatening implications
Most frequent side effects
Patient teaching

H_2-Receptor Antagonists (H_2RA)

The Wrestling Federation Presents
H_2-Receptor Antagonist Smack Down!

Zantac, Axid, Pepcid, & Tagamet **VS** Painful Duodenal Ulcer and Burny Gastroesophageal Reflux

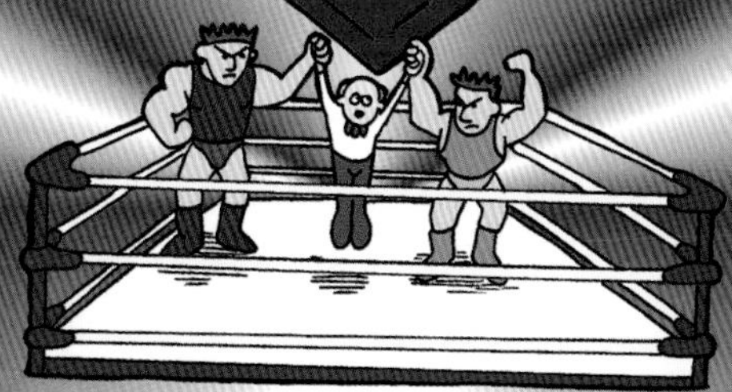

All Proceeds Will Go for the Reduction of Basal Gastric Acid Release.

Decrease in stomach acid, which may increase growth of *Candida* and bacteria in the stomach.

CJMILLER

What You Need to Know

H_2-RECEPTOR ANTAGONISTS (H_2RA)

Types

Cimetidine (Tagamet), ranitidine (Zantac), famotidine (Pepcid), nizatidine (Axid). *Note the "tidine" ending in all the generic names.*

Actions

H_2-receptor antagonists (H_2RA) inhibit histamine action on H_2-receptors, which are found on the gastric parietal cells. This action reduces the secretion of gastric acid, as well as hydrogen ion concentration.

Uses

- Prevention and treatment of gastric and duodenal ulcers
- Heartburn, acid indigestion, and gastroesophageal reflux disease

Contraindications and Precautions

- Caution with hepatic and renal dysfunction
- Caution in older adult patients
- Antacids can decrease absorption, especially with cimetidine
- Cimetidine has many drug interactions, which limit its use

Side Effects

- Diarrhea, constipation
- Older adults: confusion, agitation
- Decrease in stomach acid may increase growth of *Candida* and bacteria in stomach, resulting in increased risk for pneumonia
- Cimetidine: May bind with androgens to cause gynecomastia and impotence; effects reverse after medication is withdrawn; when given IV bolus may cause hypotension and dysrhythmias

Nursing Implications

1. Oral medications may be taken without regard to meals.
2. At least 1 hour should separate the administration of antacids and cimetidine.
3. Teach patient to avoid alcohol.
4. Smoking may decrease effectiveness.
5. Teach patient the signs of gastric bleeding (black tarry stools, "coffee-grounds" vomitus) and to notify health care provider if any occur.
6. Teach patient to notify health care provider for any indication of respiratory problems.
7. Teach patient that 5 to 6 small meals a day may be preferable to 3 large meals a day.

PSYLLIUM (METAMUCIL)

Fecal product begins to form.
Psyllium
Waste
Fiber helps smooth fecal product.
Fiber
We need to hurry. We're starting to stimulate the walls.
Metamucil mixes with food stuff and water.
Fiber
Fiber
Use plenty of water. If it gets thick, it becomes hard as a brick.
This bulk fiber is great. It gathers it, forms it, and moves it out!
You can use Metamucil or other bulk fiber laxatives to form and thicken diarrhea, but watch for nausea and vomiting.

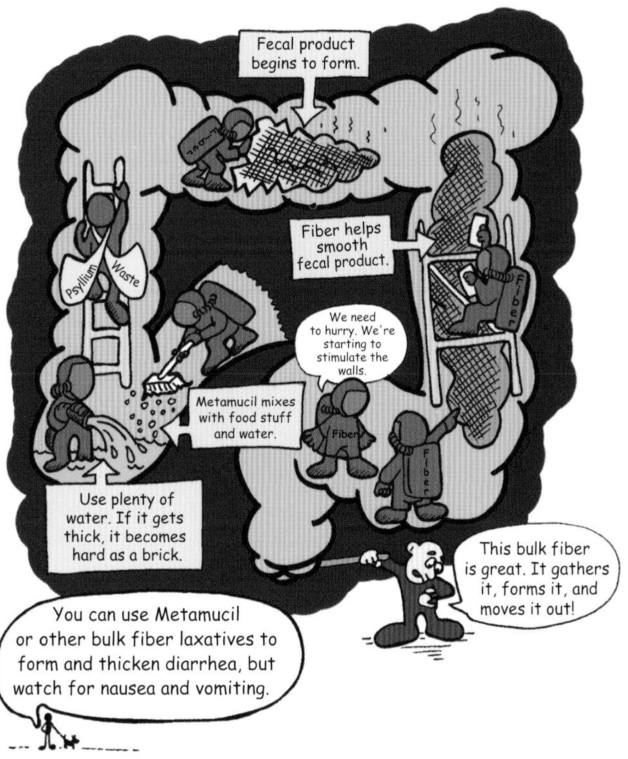

What You Need to Know

PSYLLIUM (METAMUCIL)

Classification

Bulk-forming laxative

Actions

Acts similar to dietary fiber. This medication is not digested or absorbed. After ingestion, it will swell to form a viscous solution or gel, softening the fecal mass and increasing the bulk. A fecal mass stretches the intestinal wall to stimulate peristalsis and passage of a soft-formed stool in 1 to 3 days.

Uses

- Treats constipation; preferred agent for temporary treatment of constipation
- Prevents constipation and straining after myocardial infarction or rectal surgery

Contraindications

- Fecal impaction or any condition leading to narrowing of the intestinal lumen
- Bowel obstruction or undiagnosed acute abdominal pain

Precautions

- Esophageal obstruction can occur if medication is swallowed without sufficient fluid
- Intestinal adhesions, ulcers, narrowing of intestinal lumen

Side Effects

- Abdominal discomfort, bloating
- Impaction and obstruction if not given with adequate liquids

Nursing Implications

1. Mix medication with at least 8 ounces of water; mix at the bedside immediately before administration.
2. Instruct patient to drink at least 8 ounces of water after each dose and drink at least 6 to 8 glasses of water each day to facilitate peristalsis and to prevent obstruction.
3. Bowel movement should occur in 12 to 36 hours.
4. Administer at least 2 hours before or after medications.

Important nursing implications | Serious/life-threatening implications

Most frequent side effects | Patient teaching

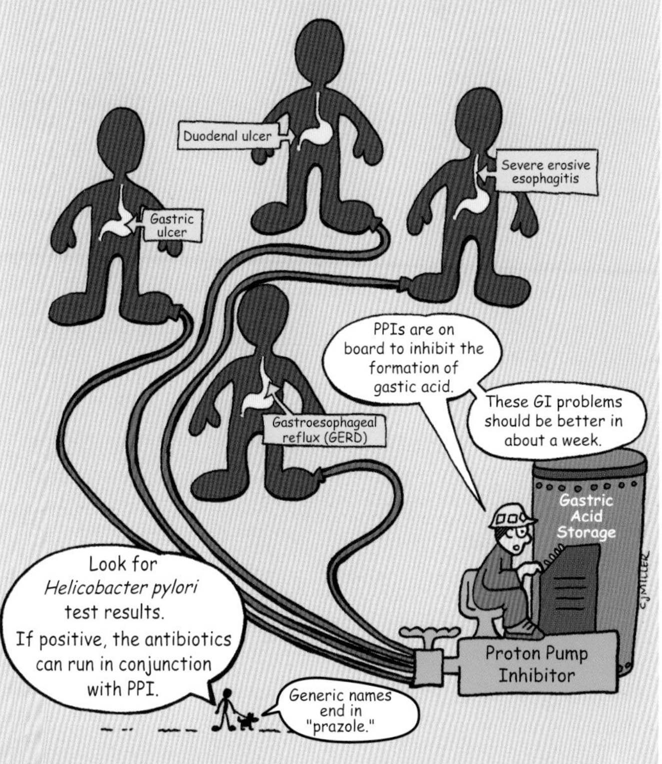
PROTON PUMP INHIBITORS (PPIs)
Duodenal ulcer
Severe erosive esophagitis
Gastric ulcer
PPIs are on board to inhibit the formation of gastic acid.
These GI problems should be better in about a week.
Gastroesophageal reflux (GERD)
Gastric Acid Storage
CJMILLER
Look for *Helicobacter pylori* test results. If positive, the antibiotics can run in conjunction with PPI.
Proton Pump Inhibitor
Generic names end in "prazole."

What You Need to Know

PROTON PUMP INHIBITORS

Examples

Omeprazole (Prilosec), esomeprazole (Nexium), lansoprazole (Prevacid), pantoprazole (Protonix). *Note the "prazole" ending in all the generic names.*

Actions

Suppress the secretion of gastric acid by combining with an enzyme on the gastric parietal cells; block the final common pathway for gastric acid formation; decrease hydrogen ion transport into the gastric lumen.

Uses

- Short-term (4 to 8 weeks): duodenal ulcers associated with *Helicobacter pylori,* gastric ulcers, erosive gastritis, and gastroesophageal reflux disease
- Long-term: hypersecretory conditions (Zollinger-Ellison syndrome)

Contraindications and Precautions

- Long-term use may predispose patient to the risk of developing *C. difficile* and GI infections (e.g., salmonella), especially in hospitalized patients.
- Long-term therapy may predispose patient to the risk of osteoporosis and fractures.
- Use with caution in hepatic impairment.

Side Effects

- Headache, diarrhea, nausea and vomiting
- Long-term therapy: pneumonia, fractures, rebound acid hypersecretion, hypomagnesemia, vitamin B_{12} deficiency

Nursing Implications

1. Instruct patient to avoid opening, chewing, or crushing capsules.
2. Instruct patient to return for follow-up if symptoms are unresolved after 4 to 8 weeks of therapy.
3. Teach patient to take medication before meals.
4. Encourage patient to maintain adequate intake of calcium and vitamin D.
5. Teach patient to report any symptoms of hypomagnesemia (tremor, muscle cramps, seizures, dysrhythmias).

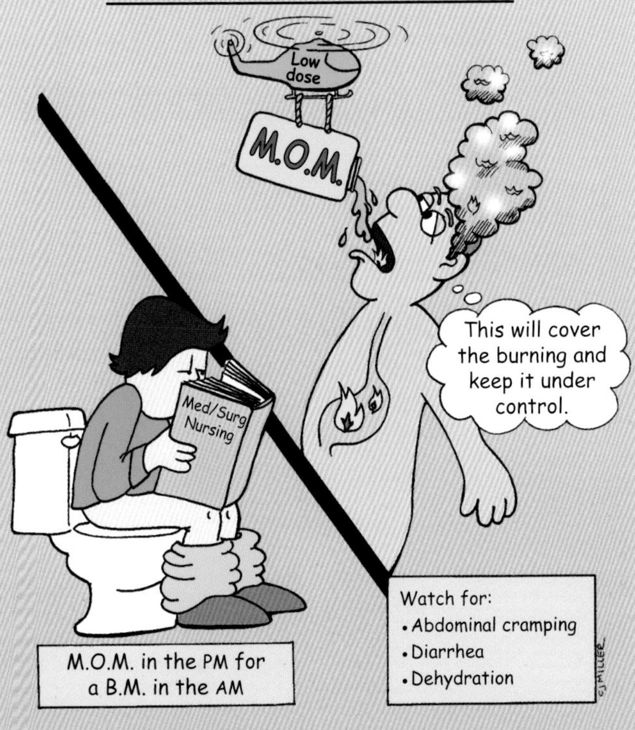
MAGNESIUM HYDROXIDE
(MILK OF MAGNESIA)
Low dose
M.O.M.
This will cover the burning and keep it under control.
Med/Surg Nursing
M.O.M. in the PM for a B.M. in the AM
Watch for:
• Abdominal cramping
• Diarrhea
• Dehydration
CJ MILLER

What You Need to Know

MAGNESIUM HYDROXIDE (MILK OF MAGNESIA)

Classification

Osmotic laxative, magnesium compound (antacid)

Actions

Draws water into the intestine by osmotic action on the surrounding tissue. The increase in fluid in the intestine will dilute the stool, stretch the bowel, and increase peristalsis. Rapid-acting antacid with high acid-neutralizing capacity and long-lasting effects.

Uses

- Constipation
- Cleanse the gastrointestinal tract
- Flush ingested toxins out the gastrointestinal tract
- Antacid

Contraindications

- Undiagnosed abdominal pain
- Renal impairment

Precautions

- Rectal bleeding
- Bowel obstructions
- Colostomy or ileostomy

Side Effects

- Abdominal cramping, diarrhea, dehydration
- Hypermagnesemia—magnesium toxicity (CNS depression) can occur in patient with renal impairment

Nursing Implications

1. Give with at least 8 ounces of water.
2. Will generally act within 6 to 12 hours.
3. Monitor bowel movement, hydration status, and electrolyte levels.
4. Laxative abuse (laxative taken every day) decreases the defecatory reflex, leading to laxative dependence.
5. Teach patient to eat foods high in fiber (brans, fruits) and increase fluid intake.
6. For antacid use, it is commonly given with aluminum hydroxide to alleviate common symptoms of diarrhea.

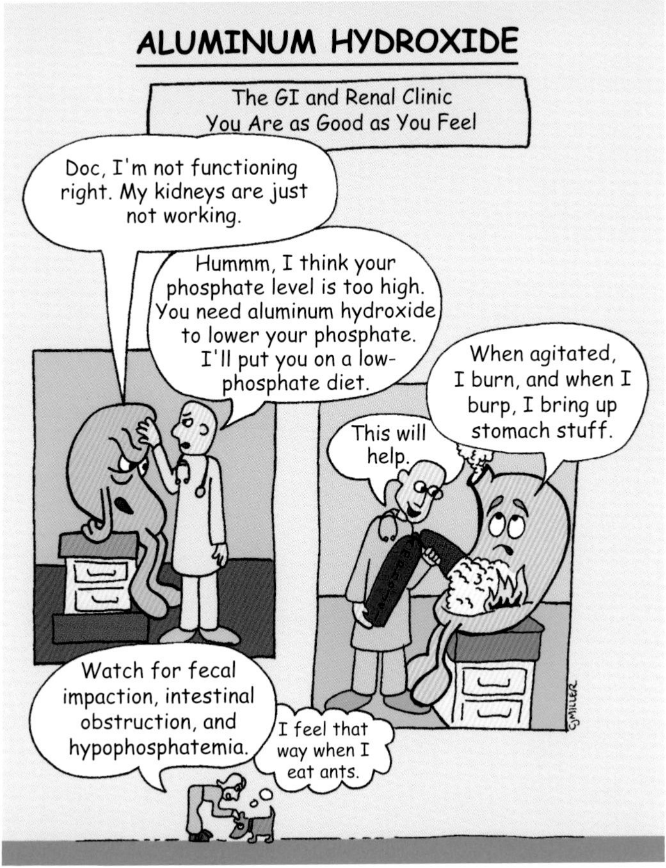

ALUMINUM HYDROXIDE

The GI and Renal Clinic
You Are as Good as You Feel

Doc, I'm not functioning right. My kidneys are just not working.

Hummm, I think your phosphate level is too high. You need aluminum hydroxide to lower your phosphate. I'll put you on a low-phosphate diet.

When agitated, I burn, and when I burp, I bring up stomach stuff.

This will help.

Watch for fecal impaction, intestinal obstruction, and hypophosphatemia.

I feel that way when I eat ants.

What You Need to Know

ALUMINUM HYDROXIDE

Classification

Phosphate-binding antacid, aluminum compound

Actions

Reduces acid concentration and pepsin activity by raising pH of gastric secretions. Binds with phosphate and helps prevent hyperphosphatemia. Decrease in serum phosphorous level may precipitate an increase in serum calcium level.

Uses

- Relieves hyperacidity related to gastritis and reflux
- Treats gastric and duodenal ulcers
- May be used to treat hyperphosphatemia in renal insufficiency
- Is most frequently used in combination with magnesium hydroxide

Contraindications and Precautions

- Dehydration or fluid restriction or both
- Renal disease or cardiac disease or both
- Undiagnosed abdominal pain, intestinal obstruction, chronic constipation, diarrhea
- Binds to tetracyclines, warfarin, and digoxin and may reduce their effect

Side Effects

- Constipation, abdominal cramps, hypophosphatemia

Nursing Implications

1. Monitor serum calcium, phosphate, magnesium, and sodium levels.
2. Do not administer antacids to patients with a cardiac presentation who complain of dyspepsia; discomfort may be referred anginal pain.
3. Teach patient to shake suspensions thoroughly before use and to thoroughly chew tablets before swallowing.
4. Teach patient to take medication before meals, when stomach acidity is highest.

Important nursing implications — Serious/life-threatening implications

Most frequent side effects — Patient teaching

ANTIDIARRHEALS

LOPERAMIDE (IMODIUM)
DIPHENOXYLATE (LOMOTIL) WITH ATROPINE

GOTTA GO, GOTTA GO, GOTTA GO, GO, GO!

Just a minute buddy. Where's the fire?
MEN
I've got to go now!

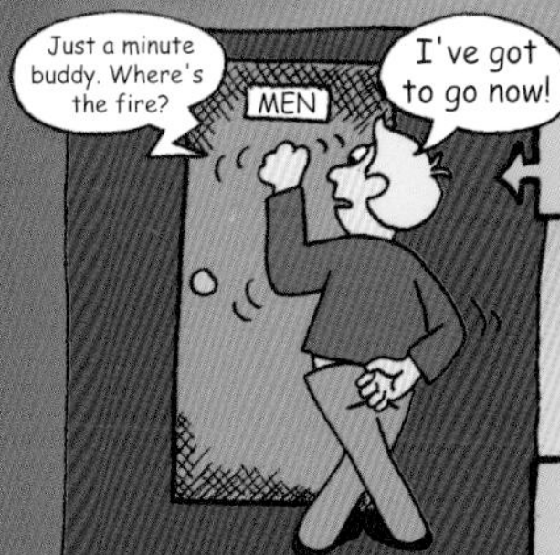

Does diarrhea always seem to hit when you are out on the town?

When mother nature calls, is it the wrong number?

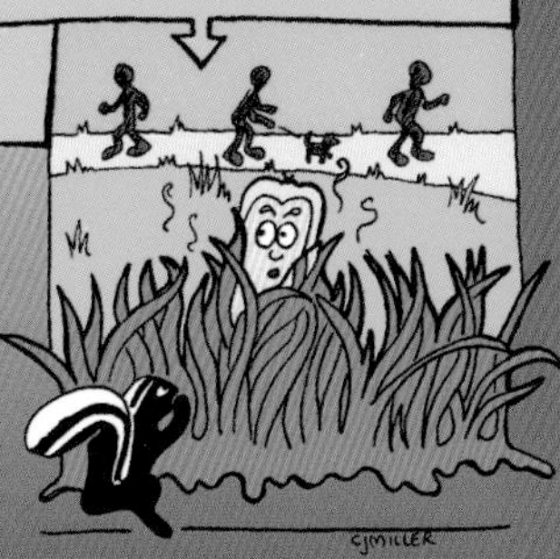

It's time to take control with Imodium and Lomotil.

Watch for dizziness, drowsiness, flushing, tachycardia, fatigue, depression, GI discomfort, and constipation.

I poop in the woods.

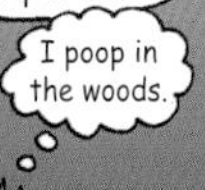

What You Need to Know

ANTIDIARRHEALS

Examples

Loperamide (Imodium), diphenoxylate (Lomotil) with atropine

Actions

Direct effect on intestinal motility; slows intestinal transient and allows for increased absorption of water and fluids. Diphenoxylate is an opioid and is combined with atropine to discourage the abuse of taking high doses to experience opioid euphoria. Loperamide is an analog of meperidine and has little or no potential for abuse.

Uses

- Symptomatic relief of acute nonspecific diarrhea
- Chronic diarrhea associated with inflammatory bowel disease

Contraindications and Precautions

- Hepatic or renal disease (Lomotil)
- Dehydration with electrolyte depletion
- Diarrhea from colitis or from infectious organism (slowing peristalsis may delay the removal of the infecting organism, which may prolong the infection)
- Imodium and Lomotil are not used in children younger than 2 years of age
- Undiagnosed abdominal pain

Side Effects

- Drowsiness, dizziness, abdominal discomfort

Nursing Implications

1. Encourage adequate fluid intake; monitor hydration status.
2. Check bowel sounds for peristalsis; discontinue and report abdominal pain and distention.
3. Do not give in the presence of bloody diarrhea or a temperature of greater than 101°F.

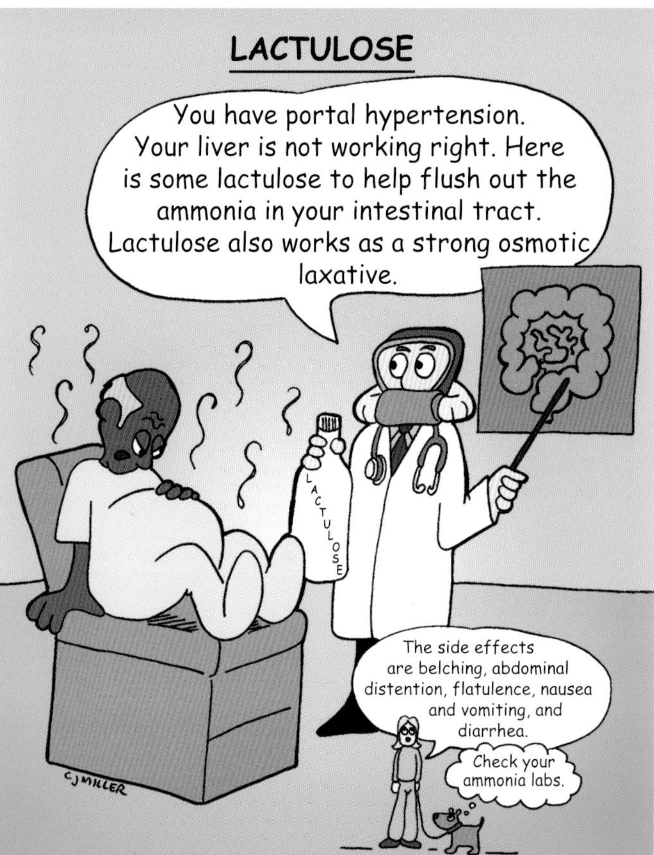
LACTULOSE
You have portal hypertension. Your liver is not working right. Here is some lactulose to help flush out the ammonia in your intestinal tract. Lactulose also works as a strong osmotic laxative.
LACTULOSE
The side effects are belching, abdominal distention, flatulence, nausea and vomiting, and diarrhea.
Check your ammonia labs.
CJ MILLER

What You Need to Know

LACTULOSE

Classification

Hyperosmotic laxative and ammonia detoxicant

Actions

Pulls ammonia into the colon from the intestines; promotes increased peristalsis, bowel evacuation (expelling ammonia from colon); decreases serum ammonia concentration in the body.

Uses

- Treats portal systemic (hepatic) encephalopathy
- Treats constipation not responding to bulk laxatives

Contraindications

- Undiagnosed abdominal pain, nausea and vomiting

Precautions

- Diabetes mellitus
- Dehydration

Side Effects

- Abdominal cramping, flatulence, nausea, vomiting
- Frequent loose stools may be desirable in excretion of ammonia; may be a side effect if used for constipation

Nursing Implications

1. Encourage increased fluid intake and high-fiber diet.
2. Monitor bowel activity; may receive dose even with loose stools.
3. Monitor serum ammonia and electrolyte levels.
4. May be given by mouth (PO) or by enema:
   - PO: Mix with fruit juice, water, or milk to improve flavor.
   - Rectally: Use rectal balloon catheter; patient needs to retain enema for 30 to 60 minutes.
5. Teach patient that bowel movement occurs within 1 to 3 days of initial dose.

Important nursing implications | Serious/life-threatening implications

Most frequent side effects | Patient teaching

ATROPINE SIDE EFFECTS

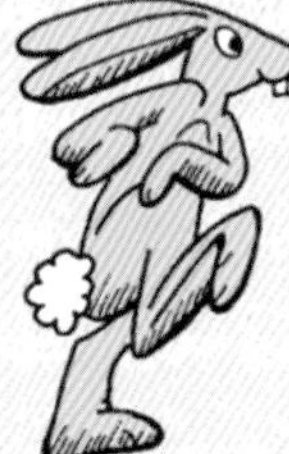

Hot as a Hare
(↑ temperature)

Mad as a Hatter
(confusion, delirium)

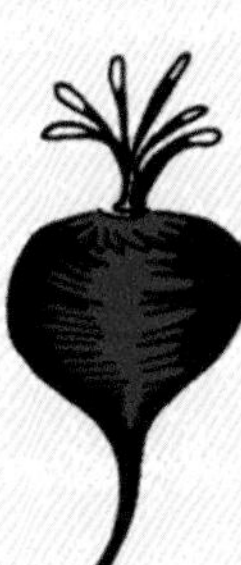

Red as a Beet
(flushed face)

Dry as a Bone
(decreased secretions, thirsty)

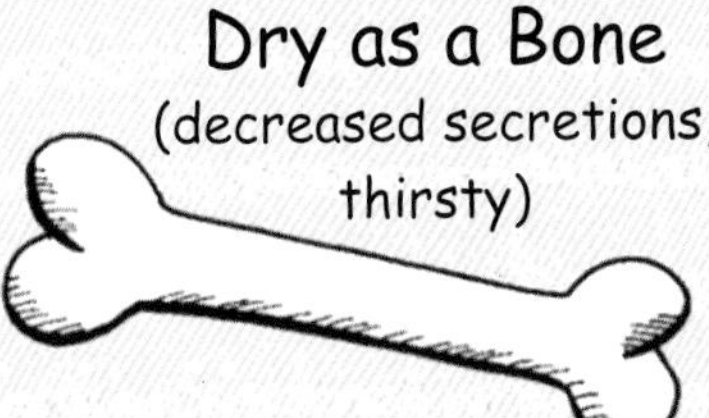

What You Need to Know

ATROPINE SIDE EFFECTS

Classification

Anticholinergic, muscarinic antagonist

Action

Inhibits action of acetylcholine. Primary effects are on the heart, exocrine glands, smooth muscles, and eye.

Uses

- Increases heart rate in symptomatic bradycardia, atrioventricular (AV) block
- Preoperative—decreases secretions
- Promotes mydriasis for retinal examination
- Decreases intestinal hypertonicity and hypermotility (diarrhea), biliary colic
- Muscarinic agonist poisoning (e.g., bethanechol, cholinesterase inhibitors)

Precautions and Contraindications

- Gastrointestinal (GI) problems—obstruction, ulcers, colitis, gastroesophageal reflux disease (GERD)
- Glaucoma, tachycardia, bladder obstruction (benign prostatic hyperplasia [BPH])
- Hyperthyroid, liver or renal disease, asthma, hypertension
- On the Beers list—avoid use in the geriatric patient

Adverse Effects

- Decreased sweating, which can lead to hyperthermia and flushing
- Central nervous system—toxic doses may cause delirium and hallucinations
- Dry mouth, tachycardia
- Blurred vision, urinary retention, urinary hesitancy, constipation

Nursing Implications

1. Evaluate hydration status; dry mouth relieved by sipping fluids and chewing sugar-free gum.
2. Evaluate frequently for urinary retention.
3. Do not administer if patient has a tachycardia.
4. If used preoperatively, explain that warm, dry, flushed feeling may occur.

Important nursing implications	Serious/life-threatening implications
Most frequent side effects	Patient teaching

POTASSIUM CHLORIDE (IV and PO)

Life Hangs in the Balance

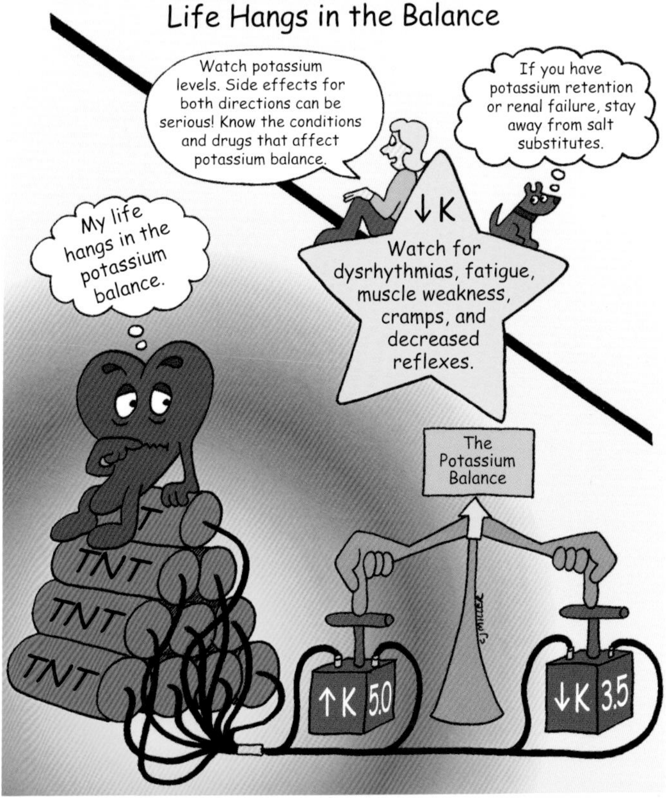

Watch potassium levels. Side effects for both directions can be serious! Know the conditions and drugs that affect potassium balance.

If you have potassium retention or renal failure, stay away from salt substitutes.

My life hangs in the potassium balance.

↓K

Watch for dysrhythmias, fatigue, muscle weakness, cramps, and decreased reflexes.

The Potassium Balance

TNT

TNT

TNT

↑K 5.0

↓K 3.5

EJ MILLER

What You Need to Know

POTASSIUM CHLORIDE (INTRAVENOUS AND ORAL)

Classification

Electrolyte replacement ▲ High Alert

Actions

Is necessary for nerve impulse conduction; maintains electrical excitability of the heart and assists in regulating acid-base balance

Uses

- Prevents or corrects (or both) potassium deficiency

Contraindications

- Hyperkalemia, use of potassium-sparing diuretics, hypoaldosteronism
- Renal impairment
- Untreated Addison disease

Precautions

- Acute acidosis resulting in potassium shifts

Side Effects

- Gastrointestinal discomfort—nausea, vomiting, diarrhea
- Hyperkalemia—(primarily from intravenous [IV] infusion of potassium) ventricular tachycardia, confusion, anxiety, dyspnea, weakness, and tingling
- Cardiac depression, peaking T waves, lowered R, depressed RST, prolonged PR interval, widened QRS complex

Nursing Implications

1. Give oral medication with a full glass of water with or after meals.
2. Sustained-release tablets (Klor-Con, Micro-K) are preferred because they are convenient and better tolerated.
3. Monitor serum potassium level (3.5 to 5.0 hr via a central lin/L normal value).
4. Watch for signs of renal insufficiency—increased creatinine and increased blood urea nitrogen values; stop potassium, and notify health care provider if symptoms of renal failure develop.
5. IV potassium *must always be diluted* before administering. **Never administer potassium via IV push.**
6. IV rate via a peripheral line is 10 mEq/hr and 20 mEq/hr via a central line.

Important nursing implications | Serious/life-threatening implications

Most frequent side effects | Patient teaching

SALICYLATE (ASPIRIN) POISONING

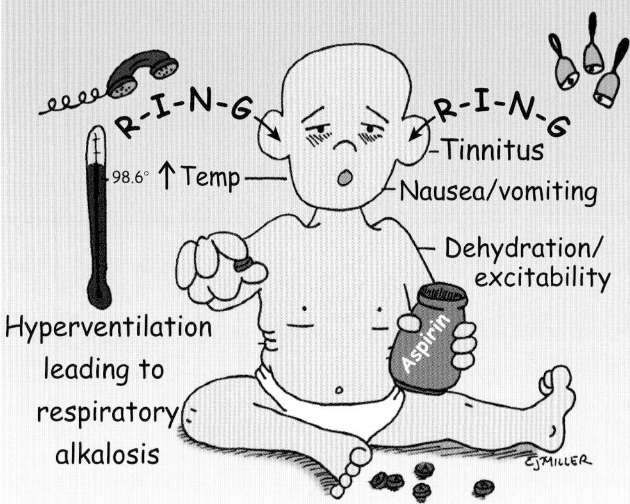

Severe toxicity =

- Metabolic acidosis
- Seizures

Severe toxicity occurs with 300 to 500 mg/kg acute ingestion of aspirin.

What You Need to Know

SALICYLATE (ASPIRIN) POISONING

Pathophysiology

Initially, respiratory excitation occurs, producing a respiratory alkalosis. As toxicity occurs, a respiratory depression occurs, resulting in an increase in carbon dioxide levels, which produces respiratory acidosis. The respiratory acidosis is uncompensated because the bicarbonate stores are depleted during the early stages of poisoning. Metabolic acidosis results from the acidity of aspirin, along with an increased production of lactic and pyruvic acids.

Signs and Symptoms

- Initial symptoms: tinnitus, sweating, headache, and dizziness
- Toxicity: hyperthermia, sweating, and dehydration; respiratory depression, resulting in respiratory acidosis, stupor, and coma
  - Lethal dose for adults is 20 to 25 g; as little as 4000 mg (4 g) can be lethal for a child
  - Severe toxicity occurs with 300 to 500 mg/kg
  - Chronic ingestion (i.e., greater than 100 mg/kg/day for greater than 2 days) can be more serious than acute ingestion

Treatment

- Decrease gastrointestinal (GI) absorption—gastric lavage and activated charcoal.
- Provide oxygen or ventilation assistance as necessary.
- Treat for hyperthermia (external cool down, tepid water sponge bath), dehydration (intravenous hydration, balance pH, and electrolytes), and reverse acidosis (slow infusion of bicarbonate).
- Provide dialysis, if necessary. Hemodialysis (not peritoneal) may be necessary.

Nursing Implications

1. Teach parents safe medication storage.
2. Teach parents not to administer aspirin to children who are suspected of having a viral infection, especially chickenpox or influenza.
3. Monitor respiratory status, blood gases, and the progression of symptoms.
4. Assist older patients to evaluate the combination of over-the-counter (OTC) medications for the presence of aspirin.
5. Aspirin overdose needs to be treated at an emergency center.

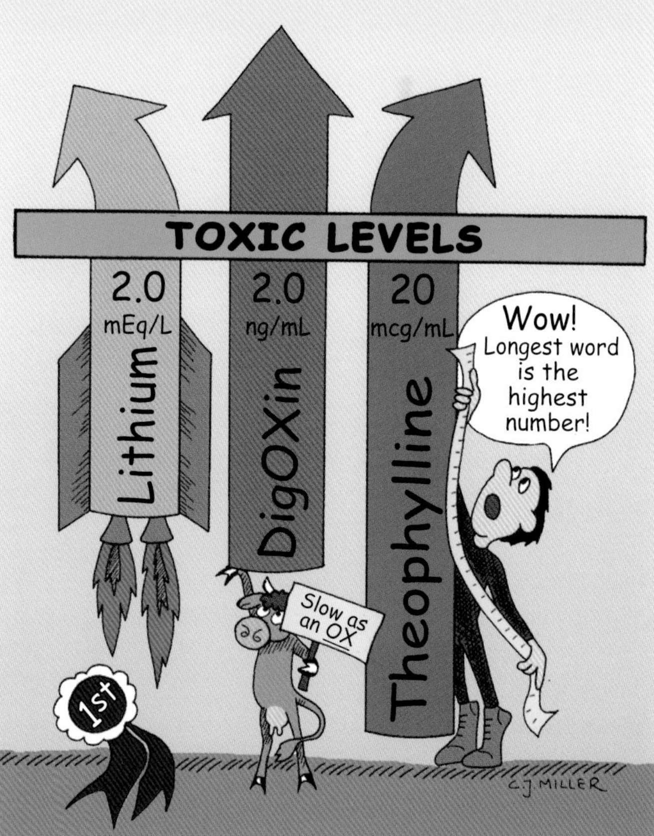
TOXIC LEVELS
2.0
mEq/L
Lithium
2.0
ng/mL
DigOXin
20
mcg/mL
Theophylline
Wow!
Longest word
is the
highest
number!
Slow as
an OX
1st
C.J. MILLER

What You Need to Know

Toxic Levels of Lithium, Digoxin, and Theophylline

LITHIUM

- Therapeutic level: 0.8 to 1.4 mEq/L; maintenance level 0.4 to 1.0 mEq/L.
- Toxic level: greater than 2.0 mEq/L (levels should be kept less than 1.5 mEq/L).
- Levels are routinely monitored every 2 to 3 days initially, then every 3 to 6 months during maintenance therapy.
- Sodium depletion is the most common cause of lithium accumulation.

Signs and Symptoms

- Side effects (at therapeutic levels below 1.5 mEq/L) include fine hand tremors, polyuria, thirst, transient fatigue, muscle weakness, headache, and memory impairment.
- Gastrointestinal (GI) effects are nausea, diarrhea, and anorexia.
- Toxic effects (1.5 to 2.0 mEq/L) include persistent GI problems (vomiting, diarrhea), coarse hand tremors, hyperirritability, and poor coordination.
- Effects of acute toxicity (greater than 2.0 mEq/L) include ataxia, high output of dilute urine, electrocardiographic (ECG) changes, tinnitus, blurred vision, severe hypotension, and seizures. Symptoms may progress to coma and death.

DIGOXIN

- Optimal level: 0.5 to 0.8 ng/mL
- Toxic level: greater than 2.0 ng/mL
- Hypokalemia is the most common predisposing factor to toxicity.
- Patients should not interchange various brands because of variations in absorption.

Signs and Symptoms

- GI signs include anorexia and nausea and vomiting.
- Central nervous system signs are fatigue and visual disturbances (blurred, yellow-tinge vision; halos around objects).
- Dysrhythmias—digoxin can mimic most dysrhythmias; if cardiac rate or rhythm changes during therapy, the health care provider should be notified.

THEOPHYLLINE

- Optimal level: 5 to 15 mcg/mL. **Note:** Use of drug has declined sharply.
- Toxic level: greater than 20 mcg/mL

Signs and Symptoms

- Nausea, vomiting, diarrhea, restlessness (levels 20 to 25 mcg/mL)
- Severe dysrhythmias, convulsions, death (levels greater than 30 mcg/mL)

DRUG INTERACTIONS & GRAPEFRUIT

Grapefruit... The juice inhibits intestinal enzymes and decreases drug metabolism...
GRAPEFRUITS INDICTED ON DRUG TAMPERING CHARGES!
Sad but true for grapefruit lovers... The juice can increase the potency of some medications.
It just isn't worth it!
CJMILLER
DON'T USE WITH US...
Ca Channel Blockers
Statins
SSRIs
Cyclosporine
Carbamazepine (Tegretol)
Buspirone (Buspar)
Saquinavir (Invirase)
Amiodarone
Benzodiazepines
Sirolimus/ Tacrolimus
Pimozide
Sildenafil
Caffeine
© 2016 Nursing Education Consultants, Inc.

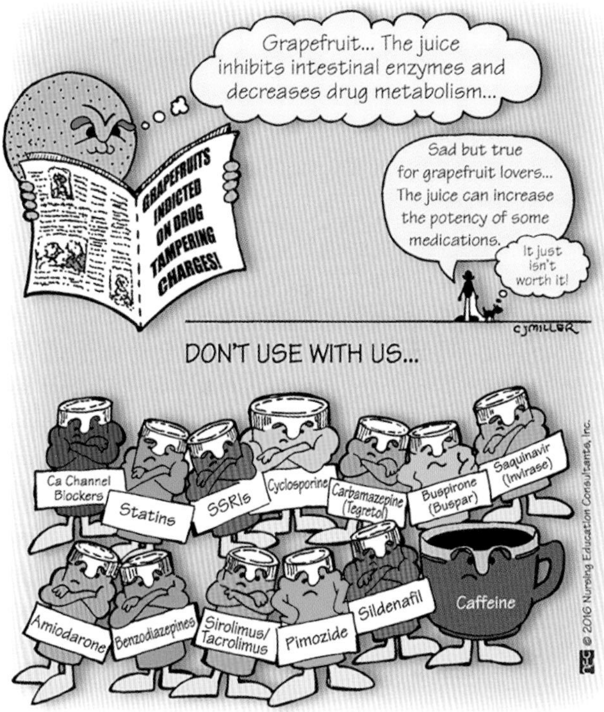

What You Need to Know

DRUG INTERACTIONS AND GRAPEFRUIT

Caution

Grapefruit inhibits the metabolism of certain drugs, thereby increasing the blood levels of carbamazepine (Tegretol), buspirone (Buspar), calcium channel blockers (diltiazem, verapamil), benzodiazepines (Versed, Halcion), statins (Mevacor, Zocor), cyclosporine, saquinavir (Invirase), and selective serotonin reuptake inhibitors (SSRIs), amiodarone, sirolimus/tacrolimus, pimozide, praziquantel, dextromethorphan, sildenafil, and caffeine.

Effect of Grapefruit on Medications

- Grapefruit and grapefruit juice are metabolized in the liver by the same enzyme (CYP3A4, an isoenzyme of cytochrome P450) that metabolizes many drugs. When the liver has too many substances to metabolize, the enzymes focus on metabolizing grapefruit while ignoring the medication.
- Because the medication is not being metabolized, it can accumulate to a dangerous level and can lead to intense peak effects.
    - The more grapefruit juice the patient drinks, the greater the inhibition.

Nursing Implications

1. Teach patient to avoid foods containing grapefruit or grapefruit juice with prescribed drugs whose levels can be increased.
2. Does not affect intravenous (IV) preparations of the medications because intestinal metabolism is not involved.
3. With cyclosporine (Sandimmune) and saquinavir (Invirase), the increased blood level that occurs with consuming grapefruit can intensify the therapeutic effects, which can lead to a good outcome. If levels rise too quickly, nephrotoxicity and hepatotoxicity can occur.

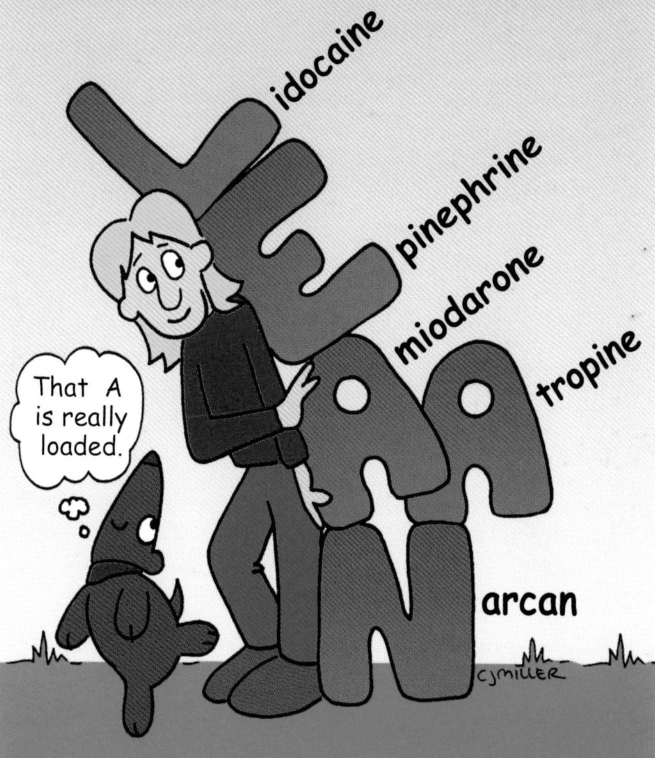
EMERGENCY DRUGS TO "LEAN" ON
idocaine
pinephrine
miodarone
tropine
arcan
That A is really loaded.
CJMILLER

What You Need to Know

Emergency Drugs ▲ High Alert

LIDOCAINE

Classification: Antidysrhythmic, local anesthetic
Actions: Slows conduction, reduces automaticity, and increases repolarization of cardiac cycle. As an anesthetic, lidocaine causes temporary loss of feeling and sensation.
Uses: Intravenous (IV) preparation only for ventricular dysrhythmias (frequent premature ventricular beats, ventricular tachycardia)

EPINEPHRINE (ADRENALIN)

Classification: Adrenergic agonist, catecholamine
Actions: Causes vasoconstriction; increases heart rate and blood pressure; is a bronchodilator; is the treatment of choice for anaphylactic reactions
Uses: For bronchodilation in patients with acute asthma; to treat hypersensitivity, anaphylactic reactions, cardiac arrest

ATROPINE

Classification: Anticholinergic, antidysrhythmic
Actions: Selectively blocks cholinergic receptors; increases heart rate in bradycardia; decreases secretions
Uses: To treat symptomatic bradycardia; to decrease respiratory secretions; to reverse effects of anticholinesterase medications

AMIODARONE (CORDARONE)

Classification: Antidysrhythmic
Actions: Decreases atrioventricular (AV) and sinus node function; suppresses dysrhythmias
Uses: Ventricular tachycardia and fibrillation

NALOXONE (NARCAN)

Classification: Narcotic (opioid) antagonist
Actions: Blocks narcotic effects; reverses opiate-induced sleep or sedation; increases respiratory rate and blood pressure
Uses: Reverses overdose by opioid analgesics (morphine, Demerol, OxyContin); treats opioid-induced respiratory depression; may be used in neonates to counteract or treat effects from narcotics given to mother during labor

CANCER CHEMOTHERAPY

Adverse Reactions and Precautions

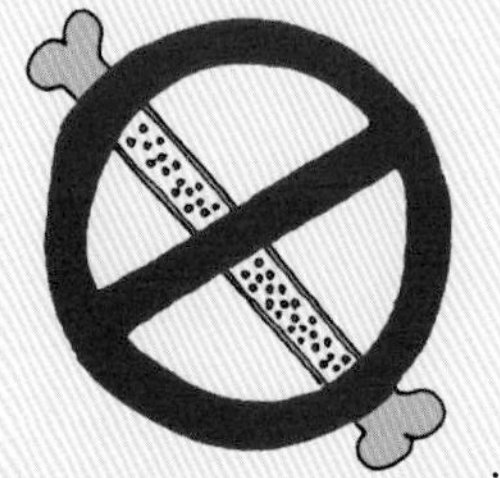

Bone marrow suppression

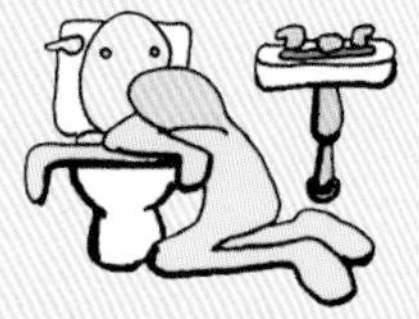

Nausea and vomiting

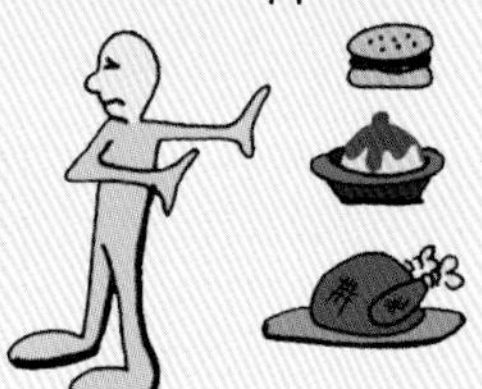

Anorexia

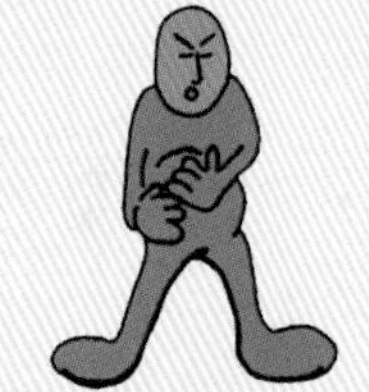

GI disturbances

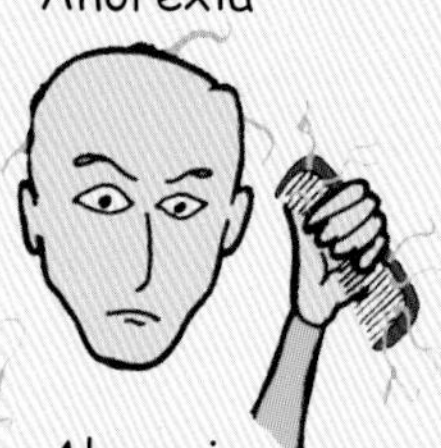

Alopecia

Avoid pregnancy

What You Need to Know

CANCER CHEMOTHERAPY: ADVERSE REACTIONS AND PRECAUTIONS

Actions

Action occurs during the sequence of the cell cycle. Anticancer agents affect cells during any phase of the cell cycle. Other drugs are effective only during a specific phase of the cell cycle. Rapidly dividing cells are more vulnerable to chemotherapy.

Dosage, Handling, and Administration

- Medication doses are individualized for each patient.
- Because of the hazardous nature of these medications, it is important that direct contact with the skin, eyes, and mucous membrane is avoided.
- Drugs are frequently given in combination to improve effectiveness of response.

Side Effects

- Cytotoxic medications are harmful to normal tissue because they lack selectivity; they kill target cancer cells, but they also kill normal cells. ▲ High Alert
- Bone marrow suppression: anemia (loss of erythrocytes), thrombocytopenia (bleeding from loss of platelets), neutropenia (infection from loss of neutrophils) may result.
- Gastrointestinal (GI) disturbances: include stomatitis, nausea and vomiting, anorexia, and diarrhea.
- Alopecia results from injury to hair follicle; regrows 1 to 2 months after treatment.
- Hyperuricemia may cause renal injury secondary to a deposit of urate crystals.
- Reproductive toxicity: fetus is susceptible to injury and malformation.
- Local injury may occur from extravasation of the anticancer drug.

Nursing Implications

1. Monitor for bone marrow suppression; may require an alteration of medication dose.
2. Side effects are expected, and patient is frequently taught how to manage the problems.
3. Observe closely for signs of infection.
4. Routine laboratory blood tests are extremely important.

ORAL CALCIUM SUPPLEMENTS

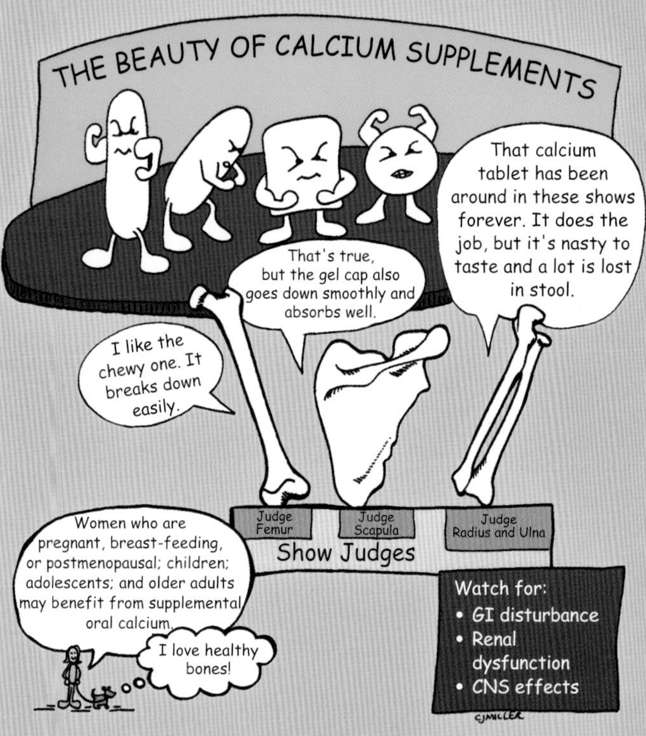

What You Need to Know

ORAL CALCIUM SUPPLEMENTS

Classification

Calcium salt

Action

Is necessary for the normal functioning of the nervous, muscular, and skeletal systems

Uses

- Treatment of mild hypocalcemia and taken as a dietary supplement
- Prophylactic for osteoporosis

Contraindications and Precautions

- Hypercalcemia, hypophosphatemia, dehydration
- Presence or history of renal calculi or renal impairment

Side Effects

- Gastrointestinal (GI) disturbances (nausea, vomiting, constipation)
- Renal dysfunction (polyuria, stones)
- Central nervous system (CNS) effects (lethargy, depression)
- Hypercalcemia—cardiac dysrhythmias and deposition of calcium into soft tissue

Nursing Implications

1. Encourage fluids with medication. Take with or after meals to promote absorption.
2. Increase fiber-containing foods to decrease constipation. Avoid foods that suppress calcium absorption—spinach, Swiss chard, beets, bran, whole-grain cereals.
3. Encourage patient to check with health care provider regarding calcium and cardiac medications.
4. Calcium carbonate has the highest percentage of calcium; however, calcium citrate preparations are more completely absorbed.
5. To maintain adequate absorption and decrease the loss of calcium, the patient should not take more than 600 mg at one time.
6. A calcium supplement is not a treatment for osteoporosis, but a preventive measure to promote bone health.
7. Advise patient against switching to different calcium preparations, as they differ with respect to amount of elemental calcium.

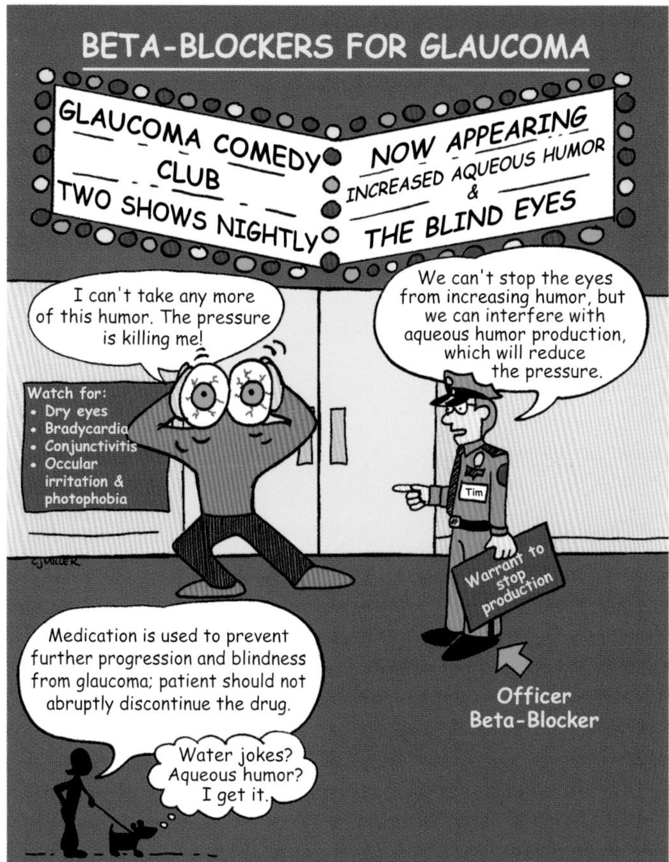
BETA-BLOCKERS FOR GLAUCOMA
GLAUCOMA COMEDY CLUB
TWO SHOWS NIGHTLY
NOW APPEARING
INCREASED AQUEOUS HUMOR
&
THE BLIND EYES
I can't take any more of this humor. The pressure is killing me!
We can't stop the eyes from increasing humor, but we can interfere with aqueous humor production, which will reduce the pressure.
Watch for:
• Dry eyes
• Bradycardia
• Conjunctivitis
• Occular irritation & photophobia
Tim
Warrant to stop production
Officer Beta-Blocker
Medication is used to prevent further progression and blindness from glaucoma; patient should not abruptly discontinue the drug.
Water jokes? Aqueous humor? I get it.

What You Need to Know

BETA-BLOCKING DRUGS FOR GLAUCOMA

Examples

Five are approved for glaucoma: betaxolol (Betoptic), timolol (Timoptic), carteolol (Ocupress), levobunolol (Betagan), metipranolol (OptiPranolol)
Note: Beta-blocker generic names end in "olol."

Classification

Beta-adrenergic blocking agents

Actions

Is most commonly used as an ophthalmic gel or drops to reduce production of aqueous humor and thereby promote a decrease in intraocular pressure. When systemically absorbed, blockage of beta$_1$-receptors may cause bradycardia; blockage of beta$_2$-receptors in the lung may cause bronchospasm.

Uses

- Primary open-angle glaucoma (POAG)

Contraindications

- Severe bradycardia, greater than first-degree heart block, hypotension

Precautions

- Impaired cardiac function, asthma or air-flow limitations

Side Effects

- Decreased visual acuity, ocular burning, conjunctivitis, photophobia
- Eyelid twitching
- Possible bradycardia and pulmonary implications if medication is absorbed systemically

Nursing Implications

1. Check patient's medical history for chronic systemic diseases that may be associated with the eye disorder.
2. Assess patient for systemic absorption of medication (bradycardia, hypotension). Instilling 1 gtt of 0.5% timolol in each eye can produce the same blood level as taking 10 mg of timolol PO (usual starting dose for hypertension).
3. Teach patient to apply slight pressure at the inner canthus for 1 minute after instillation to decrease the systemic absorption of the medication.
4. Teach patient about spacing out eye drops by 5 to 15 minutes if multiple ones need to be instilled in the same eye in order to prevent dilution.
5. Patient should avoid OTC nasal decongestants or cold preparations.

PYRIDOXINE (VITAMIN B_6) ISONIAZID (INH) AND LEVODOPA

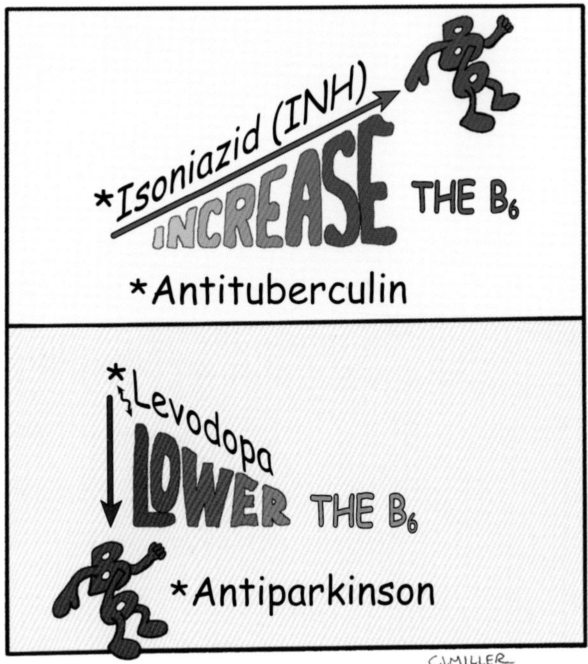

What You Need to Know

PYRIDOXINE (VITAMIN B_6): ISONIAZID (INH) AND LEVODOPA

Classification

Vitamin B_6 is a member of the vitamin B complex of water-soluble vitamins.

Action

Functions as a coenzyme in the metabolism of amino acids and proteins; it must be converted to an active form of pyridoxal phosphate.

Deficiencies

- Are common among alcoholics.
- Isoniazid (INH) prevents conversion to active form.
- Symptoms of deficiency include peripheral neuritis, dermatitis, seborrheic dermatitis, depression, and confusion.

Drug Interactions

- Vitamin B_6 interferes with the utilization of levodopa or carbidopa-levodopa, which are common medications in the treatment of Parkinson disease. Patients taking levodopa should not take vitamin B_6 supplements.

Side Effects

- Extremely high dose: sensory neuropathy—ataxia and numbness to hands and feet

Nursing Implications

1. Patients taking INH need an increased intake of vitamin B_6 to prevent deficiency.
2. Patients taking levodopa need a decreased intake of vitamin B_6, which reverses the effects of the levodopa.
3. Evaluate nutritional adequacy.
4. Perform neurologic checks in the patient with vitamin B_6 issues.
5. Teach patient about dietary sources—meats and fish, especially organ meats; heavily fortified cereals; and soy-based products.
6. Deficiency most often occurs in combination with deficiency of other B vitamins in patients who abuse alcohol.
7. To avoid neurologic injury, teach patient to consume no more than 100 mg/day of vitamin B_6.

SUNSCREENS

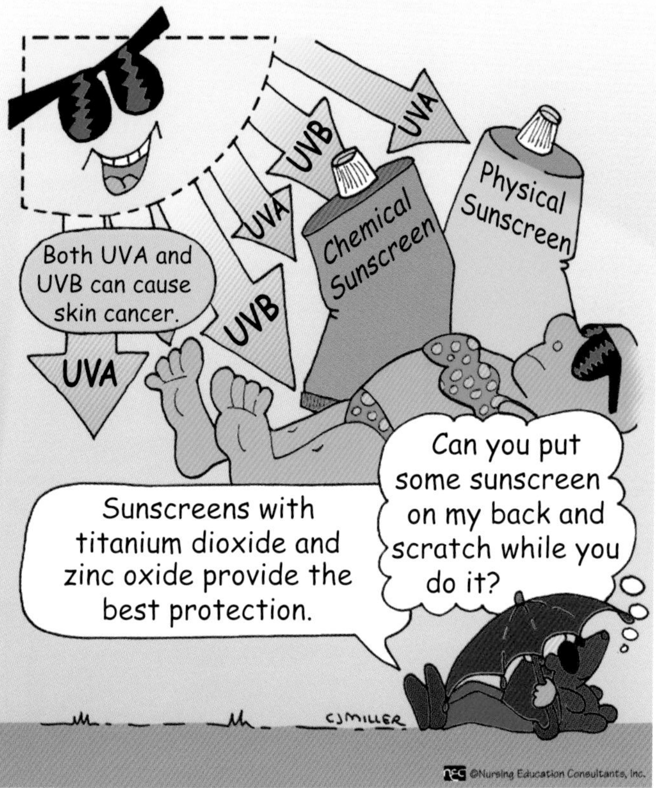

UVA
UVB
UVA
UVB
UVA
UVB
Chemical Sunscreen
Physical Sunscreen
Both UVA and UVB can cause skin cancer.
UVA
Can you put some sunscreen on my back and scratch while you do it?
Sunscreens with titanium dioxide and zinc oxide provide the best protection.
CJMILLER
©Nursing Education Consultants, Inc.

What You Need to Know

SUNSCREENS

Classification: Sunscreen

Actions: Protects skin from sunburn, photoaging, and photosensitivity reactions to certain drugs. Decreases the risk of actinic keratosis and skin cancer.

Types of Ultraviolet Radiation

- UVA—penetrates the epidermis and dermis
  - Primary cause of immunosuppression, photosensitive drug reactions, photoaging of the skin (wrinkling, breakdown of elastic fibers)
  - Is divided into UVA1 and UVA2
- UVB—penetrates into the dermis and is responsible for sunburn and tanning

Types of Sunscreens

- Organic (chemical) sunscreen. Para-aminobenzoic acid (PABA), padimate O, cinnamates, salicylates, benzophenones, and avobenzone (Parsol 1789). Most of them absorb UVB and UVA2, but to absorb UVA1, the sunscreen must have avobenzone in the product.
- Inorganic (physical) sunscreen. Only two agents: titanium dioxide and zinc oxide. Act as a barrier to the sun's rays.

Sun Protection Factor (SPF)

- SPF is an index of protection against UVB.
- Relationship between SPF and sunburn protection is not linear; that is, an SPF 30 does not indicate twice as much protection as an SPF 15.
- SPF 15 indicates a 93% block of UVB, SPF 30 indicates a 96.7% block, SPF 40 indicates a 97.5% block.

Side Effects

- Contact dermatitis and photosensitivity, especially with products containing PABA.
- PABA products should be avoided in patients allergic to benzocaine, sulfonamides, or thiazides.

Nursing Implications

1. Teach patients to use a sunscreen that covers both UVA and UVB. Read labels!
2. Teach patient to reapply sunscreen after swimming or profuse sweating.
3. Teach patient to avoid sun exposure in the middle of the day, especially between 10 AM and 4 PM.
4. Encourage other protection measures, such as wearing a broad-brim hat, sunglasses, and protective clothing and finding shade when outside.
5. Explain SPF and encourage use of a sunscreen with SPF 30.

AGE-RELATED MACULAR DEGENERATION (ARMD)

Ranibizumab (Lucentis), Aflibercept (EYLEA), Bevacizumab (Avastin), Pegaptanib (Macugen)

DRY to WET
Dry ARMD: Antioxidants and zinc help reduce the risk for becoming wet.
Wet ARMD: Responds to angiogenesis inhibitor medications.
Is it true??? They stick a needle in your eye?!!
Yes, a once-a-month treatment for wet ARMD to preserve eyesight!
CJMILLER
©Nursing Education Consultants, Inc.

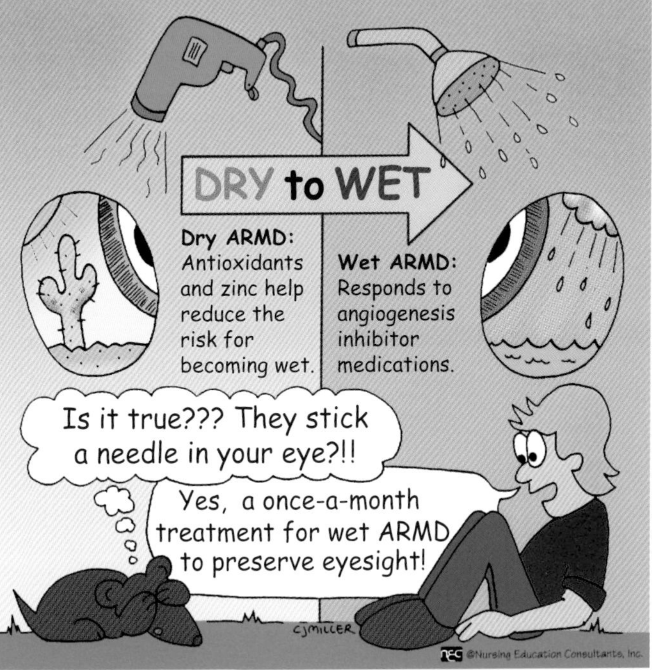

What You Need to Know

DRUGS FOR AGE-RELATED MACULAR DEGENERATION (ARMD)

Classification

Angiogenesis inhibitor

Four drugs: ranibizumab (Lucentis), aflibercept (Eylea), bevacizumab (Avastin), pegaptanib (Macugen)

Actions

Drug works by antagonizing vascular endothelial growth factor (VEGF). VEGF causes angiogenesis (growth of new retinal vessels that are fragile and leaky), increases vascular permeability, and promotes inflammation contributing to wet ARMD.

Two Types of ARMD

- Dry ARMD (atropic)—more common; less severe
- Wet ARMD (neovascular)—least common; more severe

Disorder begins as dry ARMD and can progress to wet ARMD.

Treatment

- Dry ARMD (atopic)
    - High doses of antioxidants (vitamins C and E, beta-carotene) and zinc
- Wet ARMD (neovascular)
    - **Laser therapy**—seals leaky blood vessels
    - **Photodynamic therapy**—uses a photosensitive drug in combination with infrared light
    - **Angiogenesis inhibitors**—pegaptanib (Macugen) used rarely

Side Effects

- Endophthalmitis—inflammation inside the eye caused by bacterial, viral, or fungal infection; redness, light sensitivity
- Blurred vision, cataracts, conjunctival hemorrhage

Nursing Implications

1. Teach patient with dry ARMD the importance of a preventive diet of antioxidants and zinc.
2. Monitor for copper-induced anemia caused by high doses of zinc; may need to supplement with copper.
3. Intravitreal injection (directly into the vitreous of the eye) of angiogenesis inhibitors usually monthly.

Important nursing implications | Serious/life-threatening implications
Most frequent side effects | Patient teaching

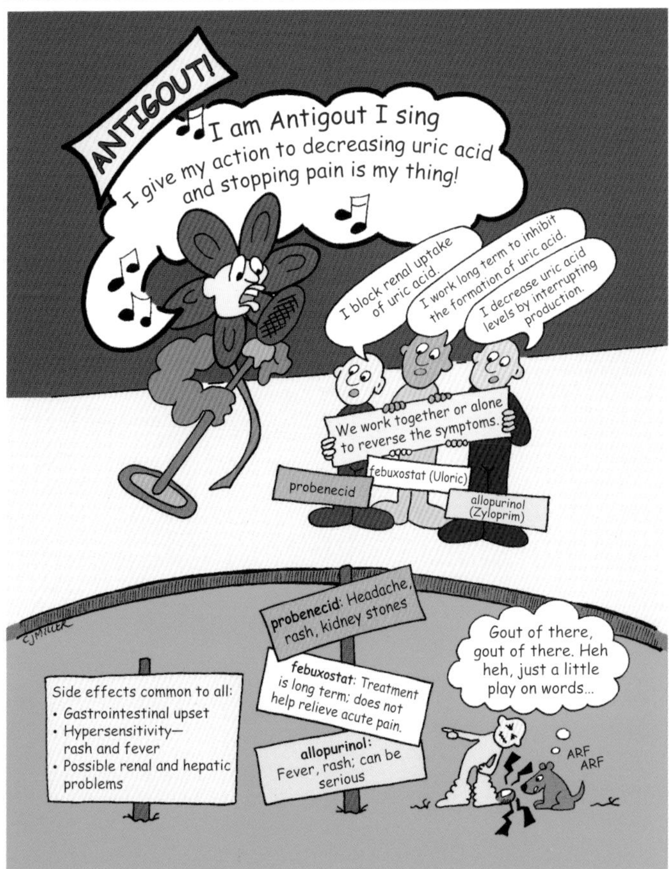
ANTIGOUT!
I am Antigout I sing
I give my action to decreasing uric acid and stopping pain is my thing!
I block renal uptake of uric acid.
I work long term to inhibit the formation of uric acid.
I decrease uric acid levels by interrupting production.
We work together or alone to reverse the symptoms.
probenecid
febuxostat (Uloric)
allopurinol (Zyloprim)
CJMILLER
Side effects common to all:
• Gastrointestinal upset
• Hypersensitivity—rash and fever
• Possible renal and hepatic problems
probenecid: Headache, rash, kidney stones
febuxostat: Treatment is long term; does not help relieve acute pain.
allopurinol: Fever, rash; can be serious
Gout of there, gout of there. Heh heh, just a little play on words...
ARF ARF

What You Need to Know

ANTIGOUT AGENTS

Examples

Febuxostat (Uloric), allopurinol (Zyloprim), probenecid, pegloticase (Krystexxa), colchicine

Actions

Xanthine oxidase inhibitors (febuxostat, allopurinal) inhibit uric acid formation. Uricosuric agent (probenecid) accelerates uric acid excretion. Recombinant uric acid oxidase (pegloticase) promotes uric acid breakdown. Colchicine used primarily for patients who do not respond to other safer agents.

Uses

- Long-term treatment of acute gouty arthritis; not useful in the treatment of an acute attack of gouty arthritis
- Pegloticase—not used readily because of significant risks for adverse effects and high cost

Contraindications and Precautions

- Severe gastrointestinal (GI) disorders
- Cardiac, hepatic, or renal disorders

Side Effects

- Febuxostat (Uloric): nausea, arthralgia, rash, and abnormal liver function studies
- Probenecid: vomiting, diarrhea, anorexia; renal deposits of urate may cause damage
- Allopurinol (Zyloprim): GI symptoms, drowsiness, headache, abdominal cramping; toxicity—hypersensitivity syndrome with rash, fever, eosinophilia, and liver and renal malfunction; prolonged use may cause cataracts
- Pegloticase (Krystexxa): anaphylaxis, infusion reactions

Nursing Implications

1. Hyperuricemic agents are given to prevent an attack; are not effective for an acute attack.
2. Initially, symptoms may worsen until uric acid levels are decreased.
3. Antigout agents can be given with food and milk to decrease GI discomfort.
4. Teach lifestyle changes—controlling weight, limiting alcohol consumption, limiting meals with meats and fish rich in purines, increasing low-fat dairy consumption, and consuming cherries.
5. Encourage an increased intake of fluids to increase excretion of uric acid and to decrease concentration.

DISEASE-MODIFYING ANTIRHEUMATIC DRUGS (DMARDs)

To Reduce Joint Destruction and Slow Progression of Rheumatoid Arthritis

Nonbiologic 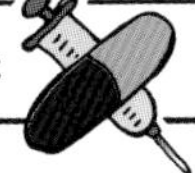	Biologic
hyDroxychloroquine (Plaquenil)	aDalimumab (Humira)
Methotrexate, Minocycline (Minocin)	certolizuMab (Cimzia)
Arava (Leflunomide)	Abatacept (Orencia)
imuRan (Azathioprine)	etaneRcept (Enbrel)
golD salts	remicaDe (Infliximab)
Sulfasalazine (Azulfidine)	Simponi (Golimumab)

Blood tests that need monitoring – CBC, LFT

Patient Education:

- Report immediately signs and symptoms of infection, bleeding, shortness of breath, or dysuria.
- Alcohol should be avoided while the patient is on methotrexate.
- The patient should avoid prolonged exposure to sunlight.
- Methotrexate must be stored at room temperature.

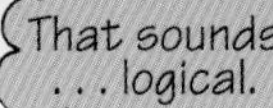

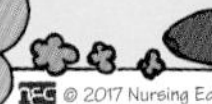

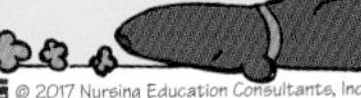

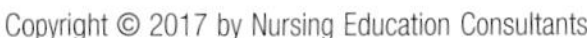

What You Need to Know

DISEASE-MODIFYING ANTIRHEUMATIC DRUGS (DMARDs)

Types

- **Nonbiologic (traditional) DMARDs:** methotrexate (Rheumatrex, Trexall), sulfasalazine (Azulfidine), leflunomide (Arava), hydroxychloroquine (Plaquenil), minocycline (Minocin), penicillamine (Cuprimine), gold salts, azathioprine (Imuran), cyclosporine (Sandimmune), protein A column (Prosorba)
- **Biologic DMARDs:** tumor necrosis factor (TNF) antagonists (adalimumab [Humira], etanercept [Enbrel]), B-lymphocyte–depleting agents (rituximab [Rituxan]), T-cell activation inhibitors (abatacept [Orencia]), interleukin-6 receptor antagonists, (tocilizumab [Actemra]), interleukin-1 receptor antagonists (anakinra [Kineret])

Actions

Reduce joint destruction and slow disease progression of rheumatoid arthritis

Contraindications

- Demyelinating disorders, severe heart failure, active infections (tuberculosis [TB], hepatitis B virus [HBV])

Precautions

- Patients who are immunosuppressed, diabetes, liver dysfunction, prone to infections

Uses

- Treats rheumatoid arthritis (usually started within 3 months of diagnosis)
- Methotrexate is first-line therapy

Side Effects

- TNF antagonists and other biologic DMARDs—serious infections (bacterial sepsis, invasive fungal infections, TB, HBV infection), cancer, hematologic disorders, severe allergic reactions
- Methotrexate—hepatic fibrosis, bone marrow suppression, gastrointestinal (GI) ulceration, pneumonitis
- Hydroxychloroquine—retinal damage (often irreversible leading to blindness)

Nursing Implications

1. Teach patient about signs of infection and to report promptly.
2. Monitor for side effects.
3. Advise to avoid live virus vaccines.

Important nursing implications	Serious/life-threatening implications
Most frequent side effects	Patient teaching

BISPHOSPHONATE THERAPY

Your days of breaking down bones are over! My squad is here to prevent you osteocasts from damaging any more bones!
alendronate (Fosamax)
risedronate (Actonel)
ibandronate (Boniva)
zoledronate (Reclast)
Those meds help maintain calcium in the bones.
Bones taste better with calcium.
BUDDY

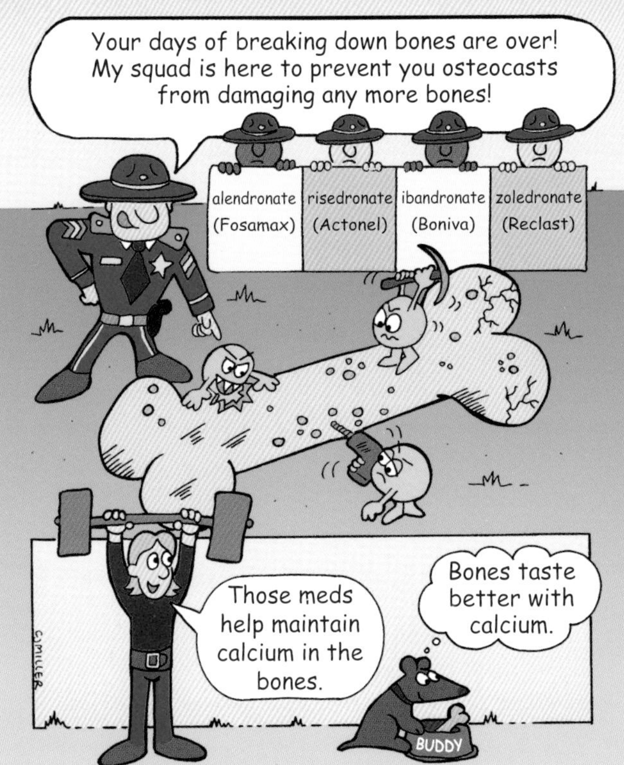

What You Need to Know

BISPHOSPHONATE THERAPY

Examples

Alendronate (Fosamax), risedronate (Actonel), ibandronate (Boniva), zoledronate (Reclast)

Note: the "dronate" ending for the bisphophonates.

Classification

Bisphosphonate, bone-resorption inhibitor

Actions

Incorporated into the bone and inhibits bone resorption by decreasing activity of osteoclasts; provides significant increase in bone mineral density

Uses

- Prevents and treats the progression of osteoporosis in postmenopausal women
- Treats Paget disease and osteoporosis in men

Contraindications and Precautions

- Gastrointestinal (GI) irritation, esophageal disease, gastroesophageal reflux disease (GERD), and renal function impairment
- Patients with swallowing disorders

Side Effects

- Oral medications—esophagitis, GI irritation and discomfort, back pain

Nursing Implications

1. Oral medications—patient should take each tablet or oral solution in the morning with a full glass of water (6 to 8 oz) at least 30 to 60 minutes before the first food, beverage, or medication of the day. Orange juice, coffee, or food significantly decreases effectiveness.
2. Patient should not chew or suck on the tablet.
3. After taking medication, patient should remain upright (sitting or standing) for 30 to 60 minutes. Patient should not lie down until after eating.
4. Patient should not take medication at bedtime or at the same time as other medications (including aspirin, antacids, or calcium supplements). Patient should wait at least 30 minutes before taking any other drug.
5. Boniva is taken once a month; however, the previous precautions are still necessary on administration.

SELECTIVE SEROTONIN REUPTAKE INHIBITORS (SSRIs)

•GET A GRIP ON LIFE•
DR. FEELGOOD'S SSRI TRAVELING SHOW!
Stop obsessive thought and compulsive activities! Get rid of depression and anxiety!
Obsessive compulsive
Depression
Bipolar disorder
Prozac
Zoloft
Paxil
Watch for:
• Headache
• Nausea
• Lethargy
• Bruxism
• Insomnia
• Sexual dysfunction
• Weight gain
Do not take with MAOIs or abruptly stop taking medications.
CJMILLER

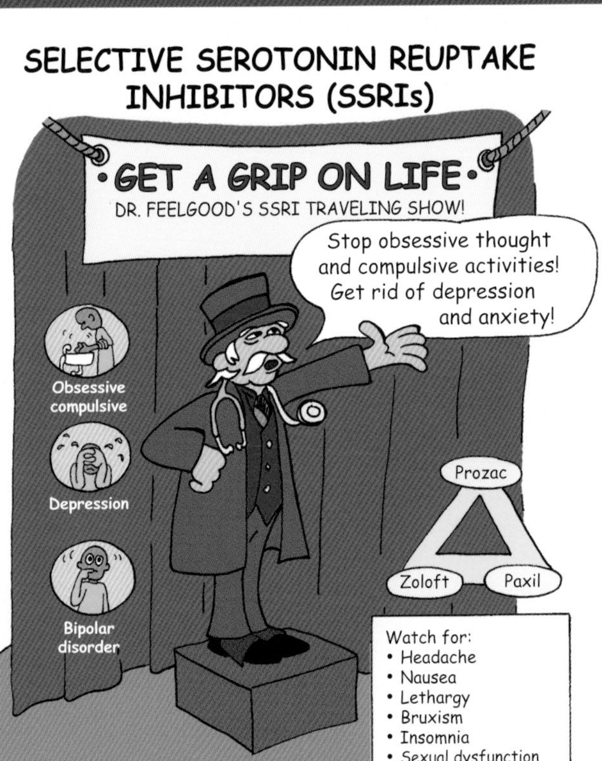

What You Need to Know

SELECTIVE SEROTONIN REUPTAKE INHIBITORS (SSRIs)

Examples

Fluoxetine (Prozac), paroxetine (Paxil), sertraline (Zoloft), fluvoxamine (Luvox), escitalopram (Lexapro), and citalopram (Celexa)

Actions

SSRIs decrease the reuptake of serotonin at selected nerve terminals in the central nervous system and increase serotonin activity at the nerve synapse. Increased availability of serotonin at the receptors results in mood elevation and reduced anxiety.

Uses

- Major depression, obsessive-compulsive disorder, panic disorder

Contraindications and Precautions

- Hypersensitivity to SSRIs
- Concurrent use of monoamine oxidase inhibitors (MAOIs)

Side Effects

- Nausea, insomnia, weight gain, nervousness, anxiety, headache
- Sexual dysfunction: decreased libido, impotence, delayed ejaculation, delayed or absent orgasm
- Hyponatremia (primarily in older adults), neonatal withdrawal, increased risk of gastrointestinal (GI) bleeding, bruxism (clenching and grinding of teeth)
- Serotonin syndrome: agitation, confusion, disorientation, hallucinations

Nursing Implications

1. Treatment of depression places the patient at increased risk for suicide; monitor patient for mood changes.
2. Do not stop taking medication; withdrawal should be gradual, not abrupt.
3. Patient should advise health care provider if she might be pregnant; SSRIs are not recommended for use during pregnancy or lactation.
4. Bleeding problems may occur if used concurrently with anticoagulants or nonsteroidal antiinflammatory drugs (NSAIDs).
5. Teach patient that it may take weeks for the full effect of the medication to occur.
6. Teach patient and family about the side effects, and advise them to notify the health care provider if any symptoms occur.

Important nursing implications | Serious/life-threatening implications

Most frequent side effects | Patient teaching

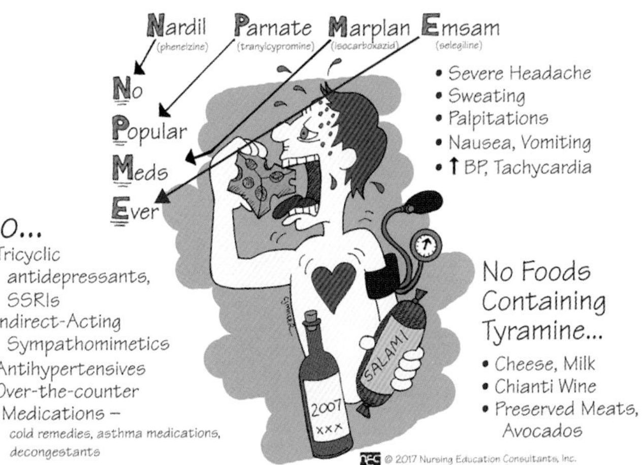
MAO INHIBITORS
Nardil
(phenelzine)
Parnate
(tranylcypromine)
Marplan
(isocarboxazid)
Emsam
(selegiline)
No
Popular
Meds
Ever
• Severe Headache
• Sweating
• Palpitations
• Nausea, Vomiting
• ↑ BP, Tachycardia
No...
• Tricyclic antidepressants, SSRIs
• Indirect-Acting Sympathomimetics
• Antihypertensives
• Over-the-counter Medications –
cold remedies, asthma medications, decongestants
No Foods Containing Tyramine...
• Cheese, Milk
• Chianti Wine
• Preserved Meats, Avocados
SALAMI
2007
XXX
© 2017 Nursing Education Consultants, Inc.

What You Need to Know

MONOAMINE OXIDASE INHIBITORS (MAOIs)

Classification

Antidepressant

Action

The antidepressant effects of the MAOIs are the result of blocking monoamine oxidase in nerve terminals. This action increases the availability and concentration of norepinephrine and serotonin for neurotransmission.

Uses

- MAOIs are reserved for patients who are depressed and have not responded to tricyclic antidepressants and selective serotonin reuptake inhibitors (SSRIs).

Contraindications

- Impaired renal or hepatic function
- Cardiovascular or cerebrovascular disease or both

Precautions

- Hypertensive crisis can be triggered by eating foods rich in tyramine and medications containing diuretics, antihistamines, antihypertensives, and ephedrine.
- MAOIs interact with many medications.

Side Effects

- Central nervous system stimulation: anxiety, agitation, hypomania, mania
- Orthostatic hypotension
- Hypertensive crisis: headache, tachycardia, palpitations, nausea, vomiting, sweating

Nursing Implications

1. Advise patient to avoid over-the-counter (OTC) drugs, especially cold remedies, nasal decongestants, and asthma medications.
2. Advise patients to tell all health care professionals they are taking an MAOI.
3. Assess patient for changes in mood; evaluate suicidal tendencies.
4. Determine if patient needs help with dosing or is capable of self-dosing.
5. Teach patient to avoid tyramine-rich foods that can lead to hypertensive crisis (fermented meats [smoked sausage, pepperoni, salami], dried or cured fish, all cheese, Chianti wine, some imported beers, dietary supplements with protein extract, soy sauce, ripe avocados, figs).
6. Patient should also avoid chocolate and caffeinated beverages.

Important nursing implications | Serious/life-threatening implications

Most frequent side effects | Patient teaching

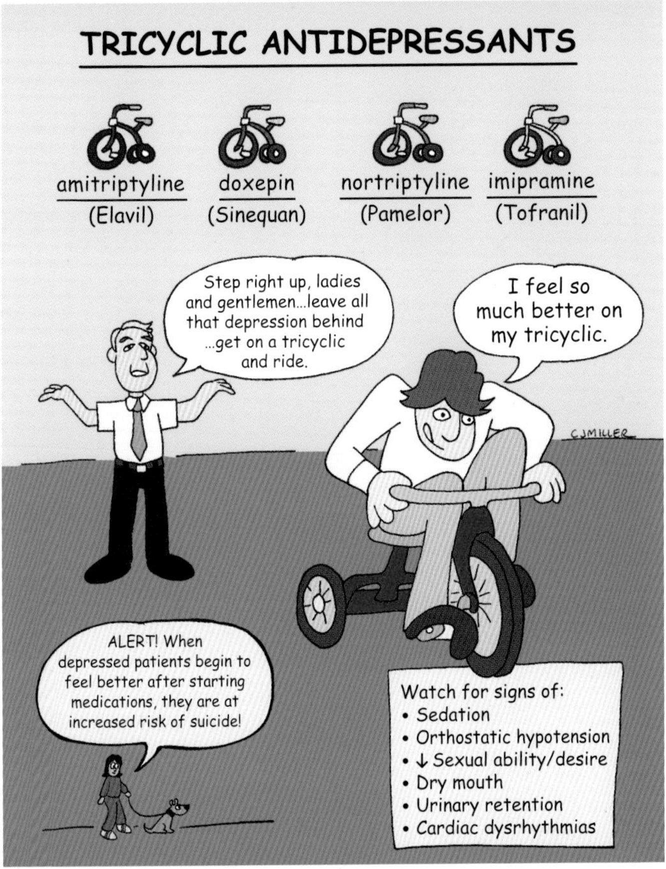

TRICYCLIC ANTIDEPRESSANTS

amitriptyline (Elavil)

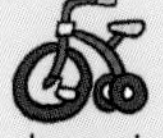

doxepin (Sinequan)

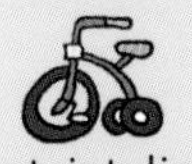

nortriptyline (Pamelor)

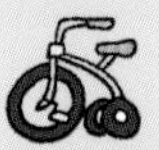

imipramine (Tofranil)

Step right up, ladies and gentlemen...leave all that depression behind ...get on a tricyclic and ride.

I feel so much better on my tricyclic.

CJMILLER

ALERT! When depressed patients begin to feel better after starting medications, they are at increased risk of suicide!

Watch for signs of:

- Sedation
- Orthostatic hypotension
- ↓ Sexual ability/desire
- Dry mouth
- Urinary retention
- Cardiac dysrhythmias

What You Need to Know

TRICYCLIC ANTIDEPRESSANTS

Action

Block the reabsorption of norepinephrine and serotonin, which allows more of the neurotransmitters to be available at postsynaptic receptors

Uses

- Not used as often as in the past; considered a second-line drug
- Depression, bipolar disorder, fibromyalgia syndrome
- Neuropathic pain, chronic insomnia, attention-deficit/hyperactivity disorder (ADHD), obsessive-compulsive disorder

Contraindications

- Acute recovery phase of severe coronary artery disease
- Not administered within 14 days of taking a monoamine oxidase inhibitor (MAOI)
- Amitriptyline is not approved for use in children

Precautions

- History of suicidal behavior or ideations
- Hyperthyroidism; cardiac, renal, hepatic disease
- Problems with urinary retention (benign prostatic hypertrophy [BPH]) or history of seizures

Side Effects

- Sedation, especially during first few weeks; orthostatic hypotension
- Anticholinergic effects: dry mouth, headache, urinary retention, blurred vision, tachycardia
- Cardiac toxicity: decreases vagal influence and slows conduction (dysrhythmias)

Nursing Implications

1. Teach patients how to manage orthostatic hypotension; notify health care provider for persistent low blood pressure or rapid pulse rate.
2. Administer at bedtime to minimize problems with sedation.
3. Advise patient to stop smoking and to avoid alcohol.
4. Therapy usually continues for a minimum of 6 months; do not abruptly stop taking medication or a relapse may occur.
5. When depressed patient begins to feel better, the risk of suicide increases; monitor patient closely for mood changes or unusual changes in behavior.
6. Beneficial effects will not peak for several weeks.

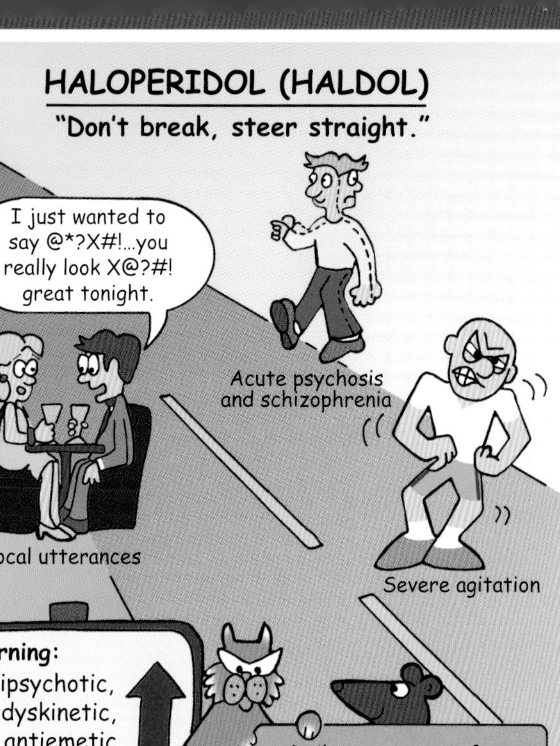
HALOPERIDOL (HALDOL)
"Don't break, steer straight."
I just wanted to say @*?X#!...you really look X@?#! great tonight.
Vocal utterances
Acute psychosis and schizophrenia
Severe agitation
Warning: Antipsychotic, antidyskinetic, and antiemetic medications needed ahead.
Daily assessments for behavior, appearance, emotional status, speech pattern, and thought.

What You Need to Know

HALOPERIDOL (HALDOL)

Action

A first-generation antipsychotic that blocks receptors for dopamine within the central nervous system (CNS), as well as outside the CNS ■ Black Box Alert

Uses

- Schizophrenia, acute psychosis, Tourette syndrome
- Sedation of patients who are severely agitated

Precautions and Contraindications

- Parkinson disease (will counteract effectiveness of Parkinson medications and increase the symptoms)
- CNS depression, angle-closure glaucoma, prostatic hypertrophy, severe cardiac and hepatic disease

Side Effects

- Extrapyramidal reactions

  Early symptoms:

  - Parkinsonism (bradykinesia, masklike facies, drooling, tremor, gait problems)
  - Acute dystonia (spasms of tongue, face, neck, and back)
  - Akathisia (compulsive restless movement, anxiety, agitation)

  Late symptoms:

  - Tardive dyskinesia (late, twisting movement of face and tongue; "lip smacking")
  - Neuroleptic malignant syndrome (rare but serious)
    - "Lead pipe" rigidity, high fever, sweating, dysrhythmias, blood pressure (BP) fluctuations, death
  - Anticholinergic effects: drowsiness, dry mouth, constipation, urinary retention
  - Prolonged QT interval and potential for dysrhythmias

Nursing Implications

1. Frequently monitor patient for reduction of target symptoms.
2. Routinely assess for presence of involuntary movement.
3. Provide family and patient education; poor adherence is common cause of therapeutic failure.
4. Teach patient and/or family member that oral liquid preparations must be protected from light and warn them against making skin contact with liquid, because it may cause a contact dermatitis.

DONEPEZIL (ARICEPT)

When It's Difficult to Stay in Touch

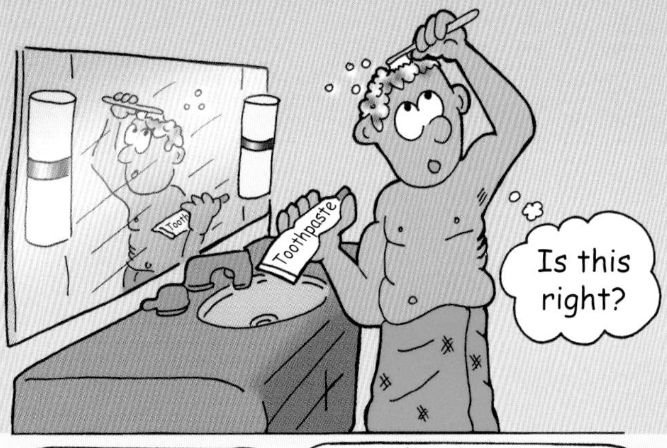

These drugs do not stop the progression of Alzheimer's disease but may improve cognitive function. Do not confuse this drug with AcipHex or Ascriptin.

Higher doses provide the best benefits but also more side effects. The dosage must be titrated... begin low and slow. Take late in the evening.

CJMILLER

What You Need to Know

DONEPEZIL (ARICEPT, ARICEPT ODT)

Classification

Cholinesterase inhibitor (cholinergic)

Actions

- Primary drugs used for Alzheimer's disease are donezepil (Aricept), rivastigmine (Exelon), and galantamine (Reminyl).
- Inhibits the breakdown of acetylcholine (ACh) by acetylcholinesterase (AChE). This breakdown increases the availability of ACh for improved nerve transmission by the central cholinergic neurons. It is selective for brain neurons.

Uses

- Slows progression of Alzheimer's disease; does not stop progression or affect the underlying disease process.

Precautions

- Patients with chronic airway problems may experience bronchoconstriction caused by increased levels of ACh.

Side Effects

- Cholinergic effects
    - Gastrointestinal (GI): nausea, vomiting, dyspepsia, diarrhea
    - Bronchoconstriction
    - Bradycardia—leading to fainting and increased patient falls
    - Dizziness, headache
- Toxic effects: cholinergic crisis; atropine is antidote for cholinergic crisis

Nursing Implications

1. Obtain baseline assessment to determine response to medication.
2. Assess for urinary obstruction and monitor for difficulty urinating, especially in older men.
3. Monitor for respiratory airway compromise and bradycardia.
4. Oral disintegrating tablet should be placed under the tongue, not chewed or swallowed.
5. Teach patient and/or family to take the medication late in the evening with or without food.
6. Explain to family that the drug is not a cure but only slows progression of symptoms.

Important nursing implications | Serious/life-threatening implications

Most frequent side effects | Patient teaching

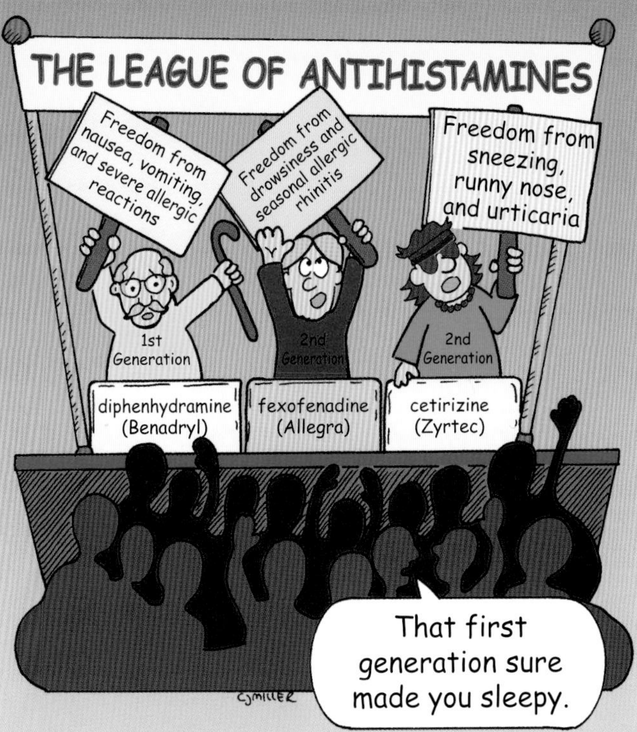
ANTIHISTAMINES
THE LEAGUE OF ANTIHISTAMINES
Freedom from nausea, vomiting, and severe allergic reactions
Freedom from drowsiness and seasonal allergic rhinitis
Freedom from sneezing, runny nose, and urticaria
1st Generation
2nd Generation
2nd Generation
diphenhydramine (Benadryl)
fexofenadine (Allegra)
cetirizine (Zyrtec)
That first generation sure made you sleepy.
CJMILLER

What You Need to Know

ANTIHISTAMINES

Actions

Competitively block the H_1-receptor sites and impede histamine-mediated responses. Second-generation antihistamines cause less drowsiness.

Uses

- Prevent and treat seasonal allergies; decrease itching (pruritus)
- Are adjuncts used with epinephrine for severe allergic reactions (anaphylaxis)
- Prevent and treat motion sickness and insomnia

Precautions

- Asthma—acute or chronic; chronic obstructive pulmonary disease (COPD)
- Pregnancy and lactation; hypertension
- Conditions resulting in urinary retention and obstruction

Side Effects

- *First generation:* Frequently cause sedation and anticholinergic effects.
  - *Benadryl:* side effects include sedation, thickening of bronchial secretions, dry mouth, drowsiness, dizziness, and muscular weakness; may cause paradoxical reaction in children—restlessness, anxiety
  - *Other examples:* chlorpheniramine, promethazine
- *Second generation:* Minimal side effects occur—drowsiness, dry mouth, constipation, urinary retention, and headache.
  - *Zyrtec:* may cause paradoxical reaction in children—restlessness, anxiety; more sedative effect than the other second-generation drugs
  - *Allegra:* certain fruit juices (apple, orange, and grapefruit) can reduce the absorption of the medication
  - *Claritin:* may cause photosensitivity reactions (avoid direct exposure to sunlight)

Nursing Implications

1. Caution patient not to take antihistamines with alcohol.
2. Caution patient about drowsiness because of safety concerns.
3. Do not administer antihistamines within 4 days of skin testing.
4. Teach patient to take with food if gastrointestinal (GI) upset occurs.
5. Advise patient to exercise extreme caution when driving or performing other hazardous activities.
6. Dry mouth can be reduced by sucking on hard candy or taking frequent sips of water.
7. Teach patient to avoid certain fruit juices in the interval between 4 hours before dosing and 1 to 2 hours after dosing if taking Allegra.

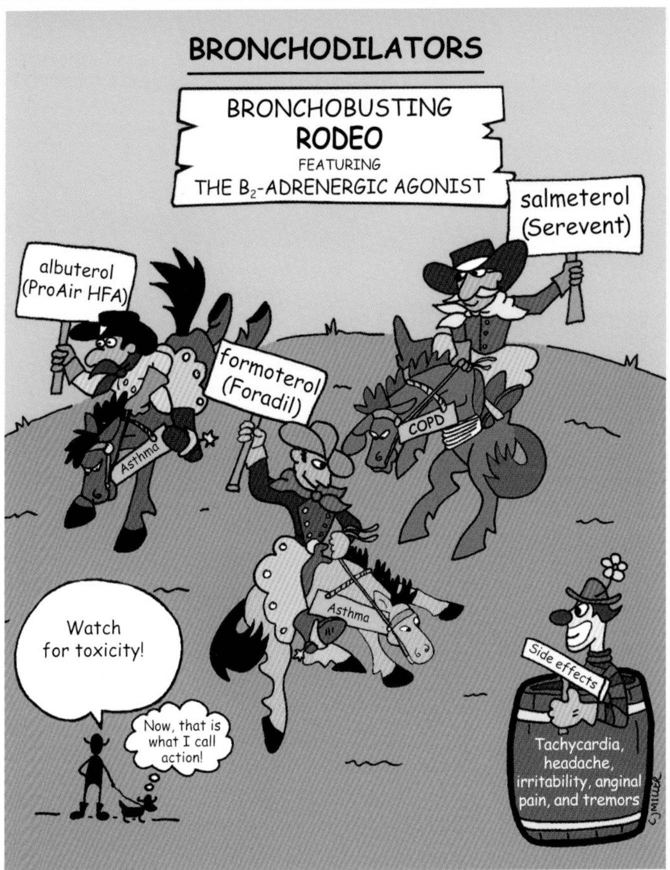
BRONCHODILATORS
BRONCHOBUSTING
RODEO
FEATURING
THE B2-ADRENERGIC AGONIST
albuterol
(ProAir HFA)
formoterol
(Foradil)
salmeterol
(Serevent)
Asthma
Asthma
COPD
Watch for toxicity!
Now, that is what I call action!
Side effects
Tachycardia, headache, irritability, anginal pain, and tremors
C.J.MILLER

What You Need to Know

BRONCHODILATORS

Actions

Beta$_2$-agonists are sympathomimetic agents that relax the smooth muscles in the bronchioles, producing dilation and relieving bronchospasm.

Types

- Inhaled short-acting preparations (SABAs): albuterol, levalbuterol
- Inhaled long-acting preparations (LABAs): salmeterol, formoterol
- Oral agents: albuterol, terbutaline

Uses

- SABAs: treat acute exacerbations of asthma; prevent exercise-induced bronchospasm (EIB)
- LABAs: preferred for patients with COPD; in patients with asthma they are not first-line therapy, but must be combined with a glucocorticoid
- Oral agents: long-term control for asthma; not first-line therapy

Side Effects

- Headache, nausea, restlessness, nervousness, tremors
- Increased blood pressure (BP), heartburn, insomnia, bronchial irritation

Adverse or Toxic Effects (Excessive Sympathomimetic Stimulation)

- Palpitations, tachycardia, chest pain, seizures, tremor (oral preparations)

Nursing Implications

1. Evaluate patient's respiratory status and vital signs.
2. Explain to patient which type of medication is for long-term control and which one is for short-term response. Short-term preparations are used to treat and/or to prevent immediate problems; long-term preparations are given on a schedule for maintenance.
3. LABA preparations are not recommended for aborting an ongoing asthmatic attack, but are used when asthma is severe and are combined with a glucocorticoid, preferably in the same inhalation device.
4. Advise patient not to use more doses than ordered.
5. Check with health care provider before using over-the-counter medicine.
6. Teach patient the correct use of inhalation devices—metered-dose inhalers (MDIs), dry powder inhalers (DPIs), and nebulizers.

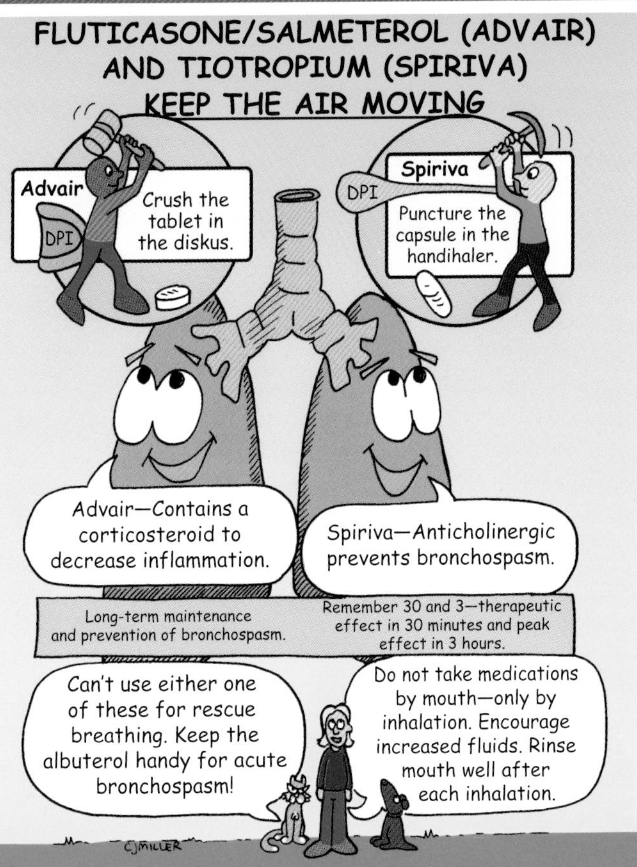
FLUTICASONE/SALMETEROL (ADVAIR) AND TIOTROPIUM (SPIRIVA) KEEP THE AIR MOVING
Advair
DPI
Crush the tablet in the diskus.
Spiriva
DPI
Puncture the capsule in the handihaler.
Advair—Contains a corticosteroid to decrease inflammation.
Spiriva—Anticholinergic prevents bronchospasm.
Long-term maintenance and prevention of bronchospasm.
Remember 30 and 3—therapeutic effect in 30 minutes and peak effect in 3 hours.
Can't use either one of these for rescue breathing. Keep the albuterol handy for acute bronchospasm!
Do not take medications by mouth—only by inhalation. Encourage increased fluids. Rinse mouth well after each inhalation.
CJMILLER

What You Need to Know

Advair and Spiriva

FLUTICASONE/SALMETEROL (ADVAIR)

Classification

Long-acting beta$_2$-agonist and glucocorticoid

Actions

Provides antiinflammatory and bronchodilator actions

Dose

Administered by Advair Diskus dry powder inhaler (DPI), one inhalation each morning and evening, or as Advair HFA with a metered-dose inhaler (MDI), two inhalations each morning and evening.

TIOTROPIUM (SPIRIVA)

Classification

Anticholinergic bronchodilator

Actions

Blocks muscarinic (cholinergic) receptors in the lung. Therapeutic effects begin in approximately 30 minutes, peak in 3 hours, and persist about 24 hours.

Dose

Administered by HandiHaler DPI in two inhalations (to ensure drug delivery of the entire contents of the capsule) once daily

Uses

- Long-term control and maintenance treatment for prevention of bronchospasm and airway inflammation associated with asthma, chronic bronchitis, and chronic obstructive pulmonary disease (COPD)

Side Effects

- Throat irritation, dry mouth, angioedema
- Corticosteroids—increased incidence of oropharyngeal fungal infections

Nursing Implications

1. Medications are to be taken every day as directed with an inhaler, even on days when patients feel they are breathing better.
2. Medications are not for rescue in acute episodes.
3. Patients should carry a rescue inhaler, such as albuterol.
4. Encourage patient to rinse mouth to decrease infection (Spiriva) and to decrease throat and mouth irritation.
5. Full effects of Spiriva make take several weeks to be felt; however, lung function improvements may occur after the first dose.
6. Teach patient how to use an inhaler.

ANTITUSSIVES, EXPECTORANTS, AND MUCOLYTICS

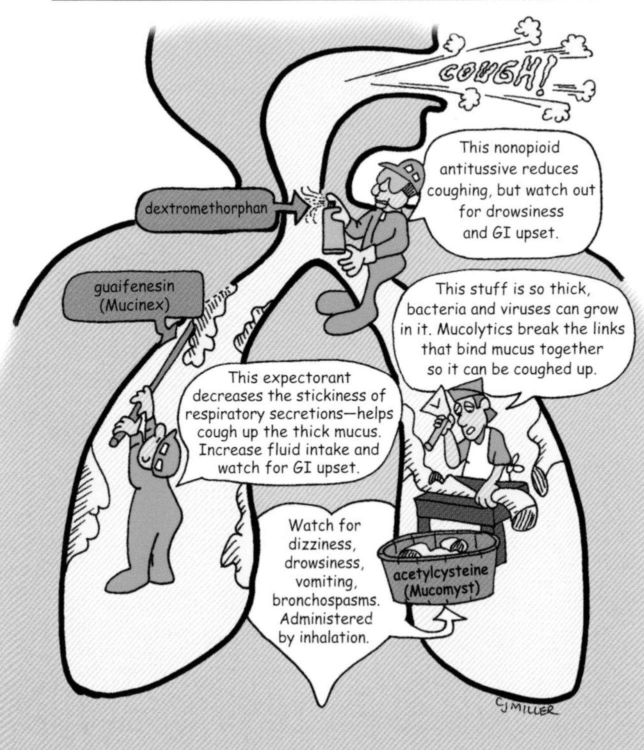

What You Need to Know

ANTITUSSIVES, EXPECTORANTS, AND MUCOLYTICS

Action

Antitussives act either centrally (central nervous system [CNS]) or locally in the peripheral nervous system to decrease irritation and suppress the cough response. *Expectorants* decrease the thickness of sputum and increase the ease of its removal for a productive cough. *Mucolytics* react directly with respiratory secretions to liquefy or make the mucus more watery, making the cough more productive.

Uses

- *Antitussives* suppress cough.
- *Expectorants* decrease viscosity (stickiness of mucus) and promote a more productive cough.
- *Mucolytics* break down mucus and make cough more productive.

Precautions

- Dextromethorphan is used in many over-the-counter (OTC) cough preparations.
- Origin of chronic cough should be investigated.
- Codeine is a very effective antitussive; is considered a Schedule V drug in cough medications and can depress respirations.
- Codeine is not recommended for children under 12 years of age or for all pediatric patients undergoing tonsillectomy and/or adenoidectomy.
- Avoid OTC cold remedies in children younger than 4 years of age.

Side Effects

- *Antitussives:* dextromethorphan—euphoria (may be abused); codeine—drowsiness, constipation, gastrointestinal (GI) upset, suppression of respirations
- *Expectorants:* nausea and vomiting, GI upset
- *Mucolytics:* nausea, rhinorrhea, dizziness, may trigger bronchospasms

Nursing Implications

1. Evaluate patient's respiratory status and response to medication.
2. Warn patient to avoid driving and operating machinery when taking codeine cough suppressant.
3. Mucomyst has a short-term disagreeable odor (rotten eggs).
4. Teach patient to read labels; cold remedies are frequently combined with other drugs and may contain 2 or more of the following: nasal decongestant, antitussive, analgesic, antihistamine, and caffeine.

DRUGS FOR CERVICAL RIPENING: PROSTAGLANDINS

Baby

Placenta

Uterus

Hey, cervix here. It's time to get this baby out of here. I need help to soften and dilate.

We are here to help the cervix to ripen. I am used most often.

Vaginal opening

Cervidil

Delivery occurs much faster when I am used, and less oxytocin is needed.

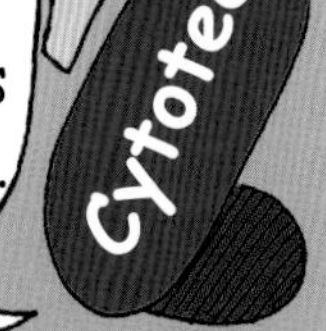

What You Need to Know

DRUGS FOR CERVICAL RIPENING: PROSTAGLANDINS

Classification

Prostaglandin

Actions

Promote cervical ripening and act on the uterus to promote contractions

Uses

- Induction of labor when pregnancy has continued beyond 42 weeks
- Abruptio placentae, premature rupture of the membranes, preeclampsia, eclampsia, fetal demise

Contraindications

- Umbilical cord prolapse, previous cesarean delivery
- Transverse fetal position, active genital herpes infection
- Placenta previa, history of removal of uterine fibroids

Types of Preparations

- Dinoprostone (Cervidil, Prepidil)
  - Gel: prefilled syringe administered intracervically by physician using an endocervical catheter; may need more than one dose
  - Vaginal insert: vaginal pouch with a long tape containing drug is inserted vaginally; tape permits rapid removal of pouch if needed; only one dose given (pouch inserted) and is removed after 12 hours
- Misoprostol (Cytotec)
  - Tablet: is inserted vaginally

Side Effects

- Nausea, vomiting, diarrhea, fever
- Tachysystole: more than 5 contractions in 10 minutes (averaged over a 30-minute window)

Nursing Implications

1. Monitor uterine activity and fetal heart rate.
2. Constantly monitor frequency, duration, and strength of contractions.
3. Oxytocin may be given 6 to 12 hours after last Prepidil gel dose or 30 minutes after vaginal insert (pouch).
4. Prepidil gel must be refrigerated and brought to room temperature prior to use.
5. Cervidil pouch insert must be frozen for storage.
6. Teach patient that she should remain supine for at least 2 hours after Cervidil pouch is inserted.

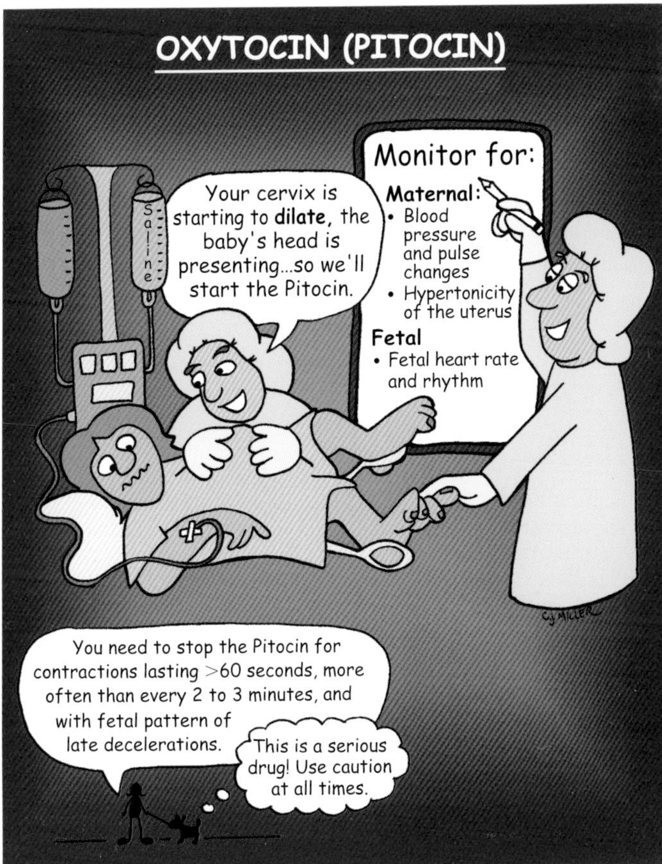
OXYTOCIN (PITOCIN)
Saline
Your cervix is starting to **dilate**, the baby's head is presenting...so we'll start the Pitocin.
Monitor for:
Maternal:
• Blood pressure and pulse changes
• Hypertonicity of the uterus
Fetal
• Fetal heart rate and rhythm
You need to stop the Pitocin for contractions lasting >60 seconds, more often than every 2 to 3 minutes, and with fetal pattern of late decelerations.
This is a serious drug! Use caution at all times.

What You Need to Know

OXYTOCIN (PITOCIN)

Classification

Hormone ▲ High Alert

Actions

Contracts uterine muscle and stimulates the milk-ejection reflex. Increases force, frequency, and duration of uterine contractions.

Uses

- Inducing term labor
- Controlling postpartum hemorrhage
- Managing incomplete or inevitable abortion

Contraindications

- Cephalopelvic disproportion, previous uterine surgery
- Unengaged fetal head, unfavorable fetal position or presentation
- Fetal distress without evidence of imminent delivery
- Placenta previa or cord prolapse, or both
- Women with active genital herpes

Precautions

- Used with great caution in women who are high parity (5 or more)

Side Effects

- Tachycardia, premature ventricular contraction, hypotension
- Nausea, vomiting, water intoxication

Nursing Implications

1. Frequently assess baseline vital signs, blood pressure, and fetal heart rate.
2. Constantly monitor frequency, duration, and strength of contractions.
3. Stop the infusion; notify the physician if the resting uterine pressure is greater than 15 to 20 mm Hg, if contractions are lasting longer than 1 minute or if they are occurring more frequently than every 2 to 3 minutes, or if an alteration in fetal heart rhythm or rate occurs.
4. Maintain input and output; evaluate for excessive water retention.
5. Do not confuse with vasopressin (Pitressin), which is an antidiuretic hormone.

Important nursing implications | Serious/life-threatening implications

Most frequent side effects | Patient teaching

Rh$_o$(D) IMMUNE GLOBULIN (RhIG) (RhoGAM)

This Rh– mom has no Rh+ antibodies, and we need to keep it that way.
You're right... this Rh+ baby can send Rh+ antibodies to mom... that's bad news for future babies.
I'm Rh+ just like my dad.
I'm Rh negative
RhoGAM
CJMILLER
RhoGAM: Given intramuscularly at 28 weeks' gestation and within 72 hours after delivery.
Stop right there! I'm here to prevent mom from developing Rh+ antibodies that could affect future pregnancies.

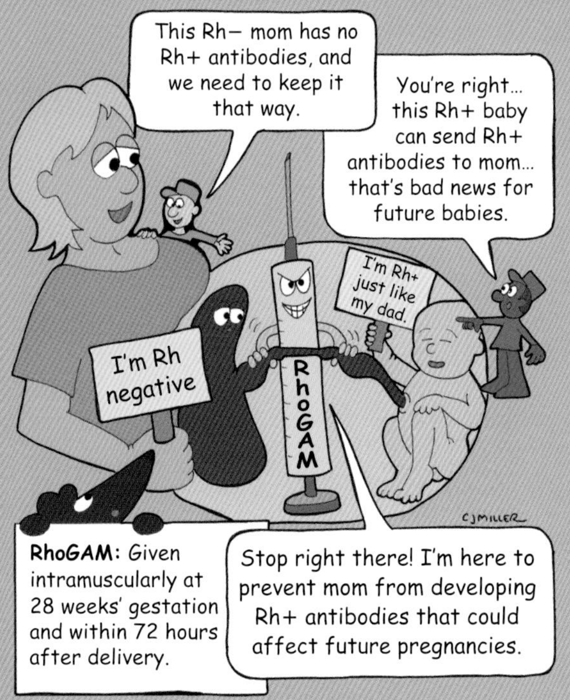

What You Need to Know

Rh_o(D) IMMUNE GLOBULIN (RhIG) (RhoGAM, WinRho)

Classification

Immune globulin; immunosuppressant

Action

Rh_o(D) immune globulin (RhIG) is a concentrated immunoglobulin preparation that contains antibodies to Rh_o(D). These antibodies destroy any fetal red blood cells (RBCs) in the maternal circulation and prevent an Rh-negative woman from developing antibodies after exposure to Rh_o(D)-positive blood.

Uses

- Prevents sensitization in the Rh-negative pregnant patient when given in the last trimester of pregnancy, as well as after abortion or miscarriage
- Following chorionic villus sampling, amniocentesis, percutaneous umbilical blood sampling (PUBS), ectopic pregnancy, or any risk of fetal/maternal hemorrhage (trauma)

Contraindications

- Not given to Rh-positive women
- Previously immunized with RhoGAM
- Not given to the newborn

Side Effects

- Uncommon
- Slight temperature elevation and irritation at the injection site

Nursing Implications

1. Administered intramuscularly at 28 weeks' gestation and another dose if delivery does not occur within 12 weeks, and within 72 hours after delivery.
2. May also be administered to Rh-negative women receiving a blood transfusion or who have had a spontaneous or induced abortion or amniocentesis.
3. Instruct Rh-negative patients to advise health care providers of their Rh-negative status.
4. Inject intramuscular (IM) preparation into deltoid or anterolateral aspect of upper thigh; do not inject into gluteal muscle.
5. Teach family how RhoGAM works, so they have an understanding of the importance of prenatal care and monitoring.

Important nursing implications	Serious/life-threatening implications
Most frequent side effects	Patient teaching

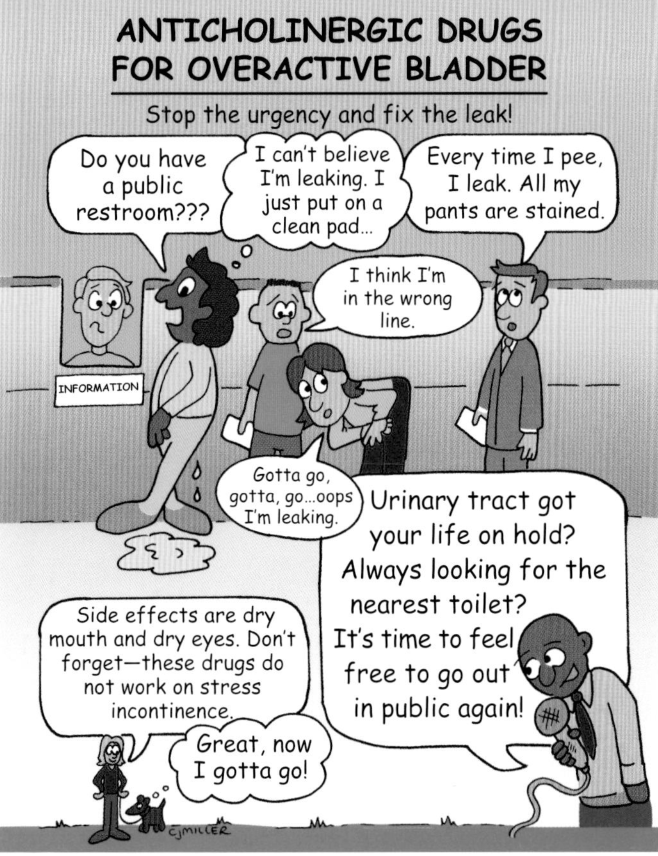
ANTICHOLINERGIC DRUGS FOR OVERACTIVE BLADDER
Stop the urgency and fix the leak!
Do you have a public restroom???
I can't believe I'm leaking. I just put on a clean pad...
Every time I pee, I leak. All my pants are stained.
I think I'm in the wrong line.
INFORMATION
Gotta go, gotta, go...oops I'm leaking.
Urinary tract got your life on hold? Always looking for the nearest toilet? It's time to feel free to go out in public again!
Side effects are dry mouth and dry eyes. Don't forget—these drugs do not work on stress incontinence.
Great, now I gotta go!
CJMILLER

What You Need to Know

ANTICHOLINERGIC DRUGS FOR OVERACTIVE BLADDER

Examples

Oxybutynin (Ditropan), solifenacin (VESIcare), tolterodine (Detrol)

Classification

Anticholinergic, muscarinic antagonists

Action

Block receptors in the bladder detrusor to relax bladder contractions

Uses

- To treat patients with an overactive bladder having symptoms of urinary frequency, urgency, or urge incontinence

Precautions and Contraindications

- Combined use with other anticholinergic medications will intensify the side effects
- Urinary retention, bladder obstruction, benign prostatic hypertrophy

Side Effects

- Dry mouth, dry eyes, blurred vision, constipation, gastric discomfort
- Ditropan: urinary retention and hesitancy; tachycardia more common; with transdermal preparations, pruritus at the application site
- VESIcare: caution with cardiac patients with QT prolongation
- Detrol: has a short half-life, needs twice-a-day dosing; can prolong the QT interval

Nursing Implications

1. Monitor for incontinence and postvoid residuals.
2. Teach patient how to use saline eye drops if dry eyes are a problem.
3. Do not open or chew extended-release capsules.
4. Teach behaviors to modify problem:
    - Avoidance of caffeine
    - Pelvic floor muscle exercises (Kegel exercises)
    - Scheduled voiding times
    - Timing fluid intake
5. Teach women the importance of using incontinence feminine pads and not a feminine pad for menstrual flow.

Important nursing implications	Serious/life-threatening implications
Most frequent side effects	Patient teaching

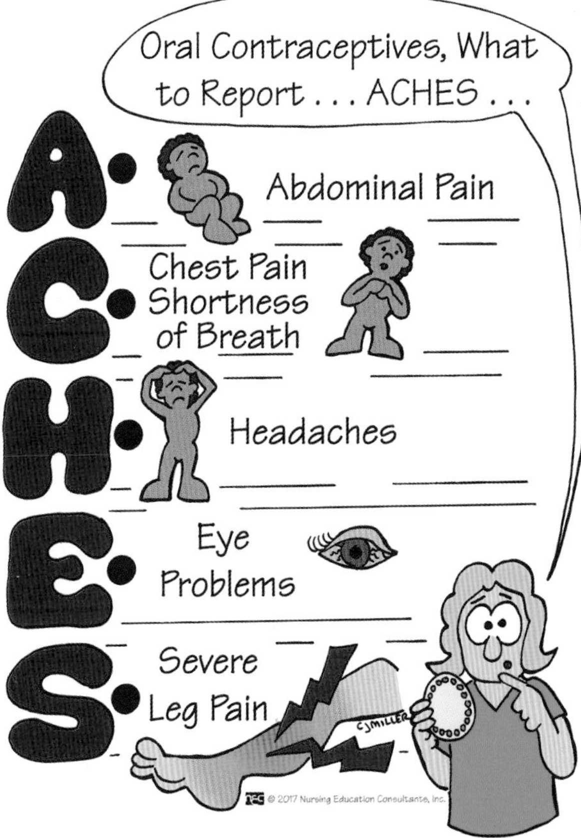
Oral Contraceptives, What to Report . . . ACHES . . .
A: Abdominal Pain
C: Chest Pain Shortness of Breath
H: Headaches
E: Eye Problems
S: Severe Leg Pain
CJMILLER
© 2017 Nursing Education Consultants, Inc.

What You Need to Know

ORAL CONTRACEPTIVES: SERIOUS ADVERSE EFFECTS

Action

Combination of estrogen and progestin or progestin-only (minipill) inhibits ovulation

Uses

- To prevent pregnancy

Contraindications

- Pregnancy, history of thromboembolic disorders, cerebrovascular disease, coronary occlusion, breast cancer, abnormal liver function, abnormal vaginal bleeding, smokers older than age 35

Precautions

- Women who have diabetes, hypertension, cardiac disease, gallbladder problems, epilepsy, and migraine headaches
- Women who are having surgery because immobilization will increase the risk of developing a postoperative thrombosis

Side Effects

- Minor: breast tenderness, nausea, bloating, edema, weight gain
- Serious: increased blood pressure, right upper-quadrant abdominal pain, chest pain, headaches, eye problems, severe leg pain

Nursing Implications

1. Patient can take oral contraceptives immediately after delivery for birth control if she is not breast-feeding.
2. Encourage an annual pelvic examination and Papanicolaou (Pap) smear.
3. If patient is using a 28-day-cycle combination product and misses a pill during the first week, take it as soon as possible and continue with the pack. If patient misses two doses during the second or third week, take one pill as soon as possible and continue with the active pills in the pack; skip the placebo pills and go straight to a new pack once the active pills have been taken. If patient misses three doses in the second or third week, follow the same instructions given for missing one or two pills and teach patient to use another form of birth control during this time.
4. If patient is taking Natazia, have her consult the package insert or a health care provider for directions to follow when a pill is missed.
5. The patient should take pills (particularly progestin-only) at the same time each day (e.g., with a meal, at bedtime). If a minipill (up to two of them) is missed, it should be taken immediately. If three pills are missed, then it should be stopped and resumed when menstruation occurs.

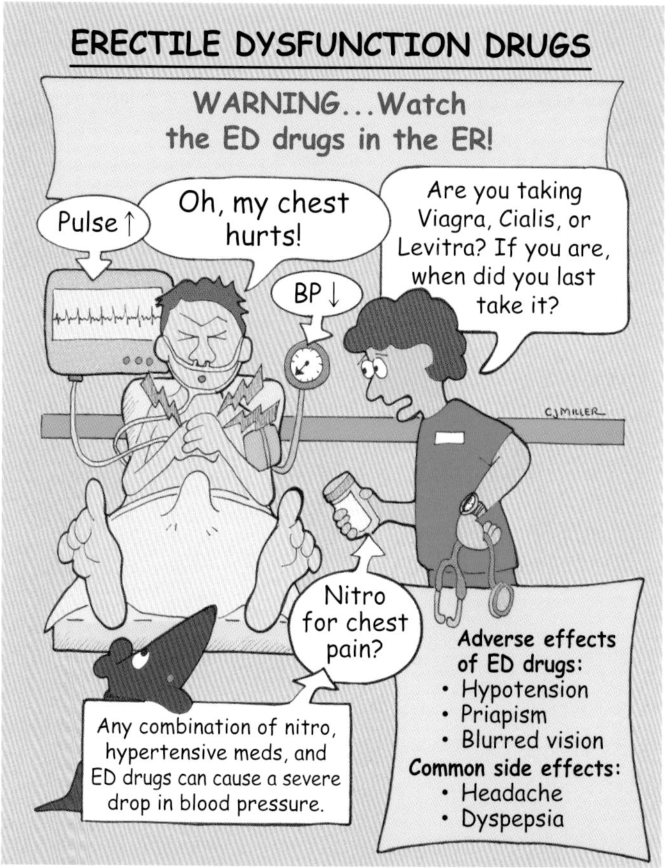

ERECTILE DYSFUNCTION DRUGS

WARNING...Watch the ED drugs in the ER!

Pulse ↑

Oh, my chest hurts!

BP ↓

Are you taking Viagra, Cialis, or Levitra? If you are, when did you last take it?

CJMILLER

Nitro for chest pain?

Any combination of nitro, hypertensive meds, and ED drugs can cause a severe drop in blood pressure.

Adverse effects of ED drugs:
- Hypotension
- Priapism
- Blurred vision

Common side effects:
- Headache
- Dyspepsia

What You Need to Know

ERECTILE DYSFUNCTION DRUGS

Actions

Phosphodiesterase-5 (PDE5) inhibitors increase arterial pressure and reduce venous outflow in the penis, thereby causing engorgement to produce and/or enhance an erection. It only enhances the normal erectile response to sexual stimuli. In the absence of stimuli, no erection occurs.

Uses

- Organic, psychogenic, mixed-cause origin of erectile dysfunction (ED)

Contraindications and Precautions

- Do not take within 24 hours of taking nitrate medication.
- Patients taking alpha-blocker medications should avoid ED drugs.
- Avoid Levitra, but not Viagra or Cialis, in men taking class I or class III antidysrhythmic drugs or drugs that prolong the QT interval.
- Dose may be reduced when patients take verapamil or diltiazem.

Side Effects

- Severe hypotension when used within 24 hours of nitrates
- Dyspepsia, headache, nasal congestion
- Vardenafil (Levitra): use caution with medications that cause a prolonged QT interval
- Erection lasting longer than 4 to 6 hours (priapism)

Nursing Implications

1. Instruct patients taking cardiac medications to consult with the health care provider about the safe use of ED drugs.
2. Ask male patients who are complaining of chest pain if they have taken an ED drug within the last 48 hours.
3. ED drugs can be taken by men who are healthy enough for normal sexual activity.
4. Instruct patient to report erections lasting longer than 4 hours to a health care provider.
5. Teach patient to report any sudden loss of vision in one or both eyes or sudden hearing loss.
6. Tadalafil (Cialis) has a 36-hour duration of action; other ED drugs have a 4-hour duration.

Important nursing implications — Serious/life-threatening implications

Most frequent side effects — Patient teaching

MEDICATION FOR BENIGN PROSTATIC HYPERTROPHY

Alpha$_1$-Adrenergic Antagonists and 5-Alpha-Reductase Inhibitors
dutasteride (Avodart)
tamsulosin (Flomax)
I PEE FREELY
BPH BPH BPH BPH BPH BPH BPH BPH BPH BPH
• Should not be handled by pregnant women (5-Alpha-Reductase Inhibitors).
• Decreases ejaculate volume.
• May cause drop in blood pressure.
Could you give me a minute? I'm no good under pressure.
Take your time. . . To decrease prostate tissue and help you pee a stronger stream, tamsulosin/dutasteride (Jalyn) are given in combination.
CJMILLER
© 2017 Nursing Education Consultants, Inc.

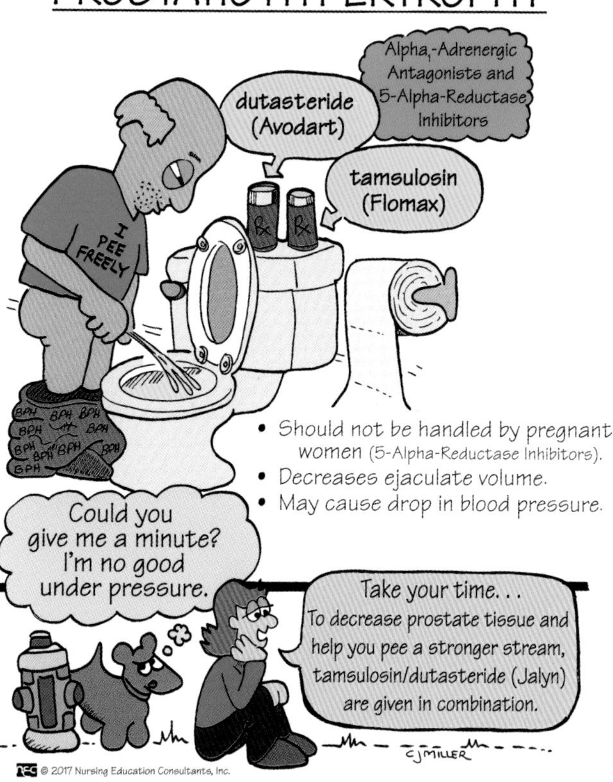

What You Need to Know

DRUGS FOR BENIGN PROSTATIC HYPERTROPHY

Examples

Alpha$_1$-adrenergic antagonists: tamsulosin (Flomax), terazosin (Hytrin), alfuzosin (Uroxatral), doxazosin (Cardura), silodosin (Rapaflo)

Note how the generic names end in "osin."

5-Alpha-reductase inhibitors: finasteride (Proscar) dutasteride (Avodart)

Note how the generic names end in "steride."

Actions

- Alpha$_1$-adrenergic antagonists—Block receptors that relax the smooth muscle of the bladder neck, thereby reducing the obstruction of the urethra. Do not decrease size of prostate. Action is rapid.
- 5-Alpha-reductase inhibitors—Promote regression of prostate tissue, thereby decreasing the obstruction of the urethra. Action is slow.
- Medications are frequently given together.

Uses

Relieve urinary obstruction caused by benign prostatic hypertrophy

Contraindications

Pregnancy and pediatrics

Side Effects

- Finasteride—May decrease level of prostate-specific antigen (PSA) marker for prostate cancer; decrease ejaculate volume, decrease libido
- Tamsulosin (Flomax) and terazosin (Hytrin)—hypotension, fainting, dizziness, abnormal ejaculation

Nursing Care

1. Pregnant women should not handle the 5-Alpha-reductase inhibitors.
2. Before beginning finasteride therapy, the PSA value should be determined and reevaluated again 6 months after therapy begins.
3. Tamsulosin (Flomax) and terazosin (Hytrin)—explain to patient he should have less difficulty urinating within a few days of starting medication.
4. Finasteride (Proscar)—decrease in prostatic tissue will take several months.

Important nursing implications | Serious/life-threatening implications

Most frequent side effects | Patient teaching

Note: Page numbers followed by *f* indicate figures.

–M–

–N–

–O–

–S–

–T–

–U–

–V–

–W–

–X–

–Z–